GLUTEN-FREE SNAC
DESSERTS COOKBOOK:

THE COMPLETE GUIDE TO GLUTEN AND
GRAIN FREE FOR YOUR HEALTHY DESSERTS
AND SNACKS. 200 EASY RECIPES INCLUDING
COOKIES, BREAD, BROWNIES, CUPCAKE FOR
KIDS.

Anna Stewart

Contents

Introduction

What is a Gluten-Free Diet?

Gluten is a protein found in wheat, rye, and barley, also triticale, a hybrid of rye and wheat. Gluten is the one responsible for making bread doughs become stretchable and binds ingredients together. For people who are suffering from celiac disease and gluten intolerance, it is damaging and toxic to the intestines. This can cause various symptoms to lower the excellent function of the gut in absorbing essential nutrients. Add to that, gluten affecting the digestive system's inability to work with a protein properly.

Barley, wheat, rye, triticale, barley, and food products made from them like cereals, bread, cookies, pasta, etc. must be avoided. In the case of oats, it is gluten-free but does make sure that it is labeled and identified as gluten-free since there's a remote possibility it is processed with the same machines used to process wheat products. Gluten can also be present as an additional ingredient in processed foods.

You may have heard about people who have chosen to go on a "gluten-free" diet, though they have no gluten-related problems. There are only three reasons to avoid gluten: you have celiac disease, you have a gluten allergy, or you have a gluten sensitivity. Gluten aids foods in maintaining their shape by acting as glue. It's also what prompts the celiac's immune system to attack itself.

The only method to treat celiac disease is to remove gluten entirely from your diet. The good news is that the human body is resilient. Once gluten is taken out from the diet, the body can regenerate and heal the small intestine. Symptoms will improve almost immediately; eventually, they will disappear entirely.

My suggestion is to take it one meal at a time. Ask yourself what food do you typically eat in the morning. It may be toasts, eggs, cereal, yogurt, or fruit. From this list, you will realize that only some of it needs replacing. Take note of that word, replace. You're not doing a total make-over. You are just replacing wheat items with gluten-free ingredients.

So, for starters, buy gluten-free cereal, gluten-free bread, and pancake mix that is gluten-free (or use the recipe in this book!). Do inspect the labels of yogurt for hidden gluten sources. More and more groceries are now offering gluten-free products readily available on the shelve easily identified with gluten-free labels. Like what was said a while ago, it is helpful to take it one meal at a time, figuring out what are gluten-free foods you are already eating, what ingredients can be substituted, and what products you need to eliminate. Some of which you can eat are actually available in your pantry. You just need to tweak something, so don't think you need to throw everything out and start from scratch!

For example, using flour for making cakes, you can substitute it with other flours such as almond flour, rice flour, or tapioca flour. Do also remember that the more you consume food in its natural state, the surer you are that you are consuming gluten-free food. Vegetables, meats, fruits, and dairy products are mostly safe to consume if not processed. The more you stick with foods in their natural state, the closer you will be to your objective.

The goal of our cookbook is to give you gluten-free snacks and desserts that your family will surely love most, especially your kids!

Chapter 1. <u>All About Ingredients</u>

Setting up your gluten-free pantry will ensure you have safe-to-eat food on hand. First, you would want to take out everything from the pantry and wipe out each shelf to eliminate any gluten. Then, toss out any open items and items that contain gluten, such as certain cereals, bread, crackers, pasta, barley, cookies, snack foods, and sauces. I recommend stocking up on the items listed below. Some may be unfamiliar to you because they're gluten-free substitutes for cooking and baking. But I assure you, these items are both affordable and available at most supermarkets.

Remember, there are many hidden sources of gluten. If you use processed foods, make sure you know what these are and avoid any questionable products. When in doubt, don't use it or check with the manufacturer first. Also, be aware that companies may change ingredients, and you should read labels each time you buy.

Foods to Avoid—Contain Gluten

- Barley
- Bran
- Bulgur
- Barley malt/extract
- Couscous
- Durum
- Emmer
- Einkorn
- Farina
- Farro
- Kamut
- Graham flour
- Matzo flour/meal
- Orzo
- Panko (bread crumbs)
- Seitan
- Rye
- Spelt

- Semolina
- Triticale
- Wheat
- Udon
- Wheat germ
- Wheat bran
- Oats, unless labeled Gluten Free
- Wheat starch

Potential Hidden Sources of Gluten

- Ales, beer, lagers
- Alcoholic beverages
- Communion wafers
- Breading or coating
- Some candies
- Croutons
- Broth cubes or powder
- Lunchmeat
- Pasta
- Prepared soups
- Prepared sauces
- Imitation bacon
- Poultry (self-basting)
- Imitation seafood
- Condiments, marinades
- Soy sauce
- Vitamin supplements
- Herbal supplements
- Prescribed medicines
- Over-the-Counter medications
- Flavorings
- Lipstick, balm, gloss

- Seasonings, spice mixes
- Caramel color

Some Gluten-Free Ingredients

- Amaranth
- Buckwheat
- Arrowroot
- Flaxseed
- Nut, bean, seed flours
- Corn
- Fava bean, soybean
- Coconut flour
- Chickpea (aka garbanzo)
- Almond flour
- Montina™
- Millet
- Potato starch and flour
- Rice, white, brown, bran
- Quinoa
- Sorghum
- Rice, sweet, sticky
- Sago
- Teff
- Tapioca

Gluten-Free Baking

Gluten-free baking is an opportunity to learn because it's one of the most challenging processes to master — it's truly a science. When we get away from a simple cup of overly processed wheat flour and eggs, we can play, becoming acquainted with a variety of fresh flavors and outcomes. Gluten-free baked goods won't taste like conventional baked goods made with wheat flour, processed sugars, and butter; they'll taste like a new world of goodness. Flavor profiles will be deeper and richer, and textures will be more natural — this is because nutrients are still intact.

Flours

Combining is the name of the game when it comes to gluten-free flours. They each have their personality, texture, and flavor, and they work best when partnered with differing personalities.

Easily make flours using a food processor (oats and buckwheat work well), and then if necessary, to get a dustier, more refined texture, use a coffee or spice grinder for dense nuts and seeds. Just make sure you don't over-process and end up with butter (which could be a delicious, happy accident if you don't need the flour). A grain mill (best option) processes grains, nuts, and seeds beautifully (and can be purchased as a relatively small attachment if you have a standing mixer). Grinding your flours also allows you to soak and dry ingredients first for optimal nutrient assimilation.

One of my favorite tips for using gluten-free flours, particularly ones with an earthy, grassy taste like quinoa and amaranth flour, is to toast them for about 7 minutes before incorporating into a recipe. Toasting rounds out sharp flavors and adds a nice richness to flour.

There are so many choices you can choose from, but after countless successes and failures, these are the flours I prefer to bake with at the moment:

- Almond Flour

Nice moisture content and texture for muffins, cakes, and bread. Blanched almond flour works best and partners well with a more fine-textured, dry flour for balance. Try it in crackers or cake

- Arrowroot Starch

Not only does this fine, starchy flour make a fantastic cornstarch replacement for sauces and gravies, but it can lighten the heavy mouthfeel that comes with dense flours like almond. It also creates a nice crumb with baked goods and helps make a pliable, gluten-free crepe.

- Buckwheat Flour

Contrary to what its name implies, this unique, dark flour is gluten-free. It's nutty and earthy in flavor and loaded with nutrient benefits. It makes great pancakes, cookies, muffins, and crackers.

- Garbanzo Flour

A creamy, dense, bean-flavored flour that works very well mixed with the sweetness of almond flour (sifting helps lighten texture before baking). Alone, it makes fantastic crepes and flatbreads. Garbanzo & fava bean flour (aka garfava) can be substituted in equal amounts for garbanzo.

- Millet Flour

A sweet, mild flavor that will work well in combinations with moist ingredients since it creates a nice, crumbly texture.

- Oat Flour

Nothing comes as close to the taste and texture of conventional baked goods as oat flour. Still, it's so important that we use certified gluten-free, especially if diagnosed with sensitivity or celiac. If you can't find reputable gluten-free flour, get oats from a trusted source and grind your own. Oat flour has a slightly nutty flavor and chewy texture that makes incredible Walnut Chocolate Chip Cookies.

- Rice Flour

Brown rice contains the nutritious bran and germ, and white rice does not (thanks, processing). Brown rice flour is nutty and sweet and has a gritty texture that'll result in a denser baked good. White rice flour is a bit more neutral in flavor with the same gritty texture. Sweet rice flour, sometimes called glutinous rice flour (even though there is no gluten present), can add necessary chew to baked goods.

- Sorghum Flour

Paired with moist flours like almond, sorghum can replicate the flavor and texture that most folks are used to with conventional baked goods. It's up there with oat flour in my book and has a sweet taste and relatively smooth texture (an almost undetectable bit of grit).

OTHER INGREDIENTS:

Leavening Agents

- Baking Powder: I use a gluten-free and aluminum-free brand like Rumford. Baking powder is my friend.

- Baking Soda: works as a leavening agent when combined with something acidic like sourdough. Great for pancakes and other batters. It also causes cookies to spread.

- Egg: just good, old-fashioned, farm-fresh eggs work great to bind and fluff things up. Farm fresh is best because the hens are allowed to roam and eat bugs, contributing to their nice orange yolks, which are high in vitamin A.

Seeds

- Flax: Awesome oil source, great for the digestive system, great egg replacer (only it doesn't whip up to make meringue-like egg white, which I think is rather sad).

- Sesame seeds: Great for making crackers and bars.

Starches

- Arrowroot Powder: whole root, not just the starch, although it still is a starch. I use a minimal amount in my cooking. None in my bread.

- Non-GMO Cornstarch: I use a minimal amount on a rare occasion like dusting homemade egg roll wraps, to keep them from sticking.

Sweeteners

- Raw Honey: super yummy sweet syrup made by bees. Despite popular belief, it has many beneficial properties, one of which is combatting or alleviating seasonal allergies.

- Agave: syrup is made from the agave plant and is also low glycemic. However, it contains fructose, which may interfere with metabolism in high amounts. Any liquid sweetener may be used in recipes calling for agave.

- Coconut Nectar: syrup tapped from the coconut tree. Very low glycemic, neutral taste. However, it is expensive.

- Grade A or B Maple Syrup: Real syrup tapped from maple trees, high in nutrients, rich in flavor.

Oils

- Butter: Great source of fat when made from healthy, properly fed cows. When this isn't possible, then at least healthy cows that haven't been injected with hormones or medications (because what they eat and are injected with goes through their milk and into you).

- Coconut Oil, Virgin, or extra virgin: antimicrobial, antibacterial, antifungal, helps thyroid function—the best oil to use for cooking because of its high heat tolerance as opposed to most other oils. A great butter substitute, whether spreading over toast or using in recipes and makes your hands soft if you use it as a lotion.

- Olive Oil—Great oil for use in salads.

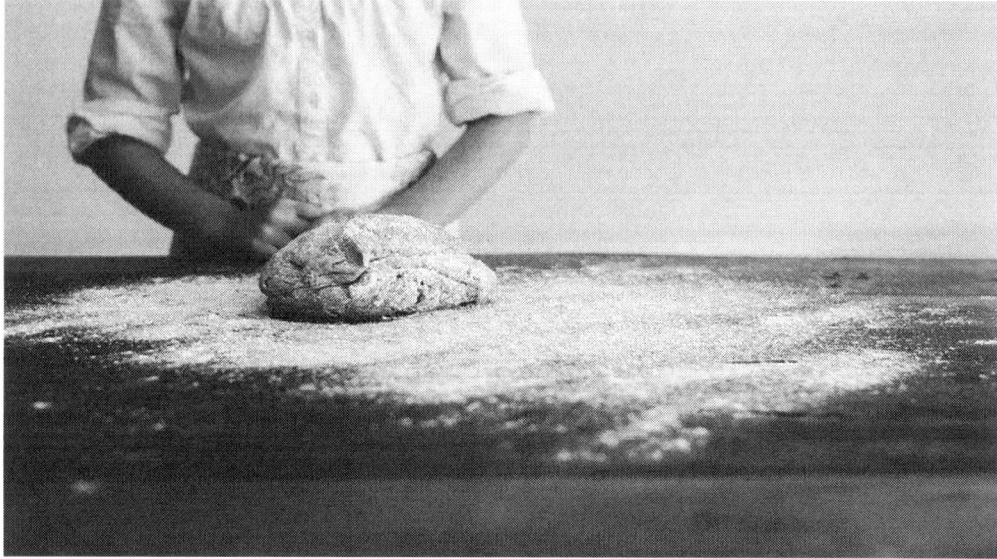

Chapter 2. __BREAKFASTS__

1. Spinach and Bacon Frittata

Ingredients:

- √ 8 oz. bacon
- √ 8 eggs
- √ salt and pepper
- √ 1 large tomato, sliced
- √ 1 cup spinach
- √ 4 oz. cheese, grated, omit if dairy-free

Dairy-free

Preparation Time: 10 minutes
Cooking Time: 15 minutes
Servings: 4
Difficult: Easy

Directions:

Preheat broiler and fry bacon. Whisk together eggs, salt, and pepper. Pour beaten eggs into a muffin pan, and cook until the center is wet. Add tomato slices, spinach, and bacon. Continue cooking. Top with cheese. Broil uuntil cheese is melted.

Nutrition:

Calories: 180 g

Fat: 8.3g

Fiber: 2.5g

Carbs: 5.4g

Protein: 7g

2. Crustless Ham Quiche

Ingredients:

- √ 6 eggs
- √ 1 cup coconut milk
- √ 4 oz. ham, diced
- √ 1 (4-oz.) can dice green chilies
- √ 1 ½ cup shredded dairy-free cheese
- √ 3 diced green onions
- √ Pepper and salt

Dairy-free

Preparation Time: 10 minutes
Cooking Time: 40 minutes
Servings: 3
Difficulty: Easy

Directions:

Oven: 325°F

Whisk eggs well. Then add half & half and continue whisking until well blended. Add all other remaining ingredients. Pour into a pan. Bake for 40 minutes.

Nutrition:

Calories: 182

Fat: 9.3g

Fiber: 3.2g

Carbs: 9.7g

Protein: 11.7g

3. Breakfast Danish

Ingredients:

Dairy-free

FLOUR BLEND (2 cups total):

Preparation Time: 35 minutes

- √ ½ cup tapioca starch
- √ ½ cup potato starch
- √ ⅓ cup brown rice flour
- √ ⅓ cup almond flour
- √ ⅓ cup sorghum flour
- √ 1 tsp. gelatin powder
- √ 1 tsp. baking powder

Cooking Time: 60 minutes

Difficulty: Hard

Servings: 6

BASE LAYER

- √ ½ cup shortening
- √ 1 cup gluten-free flour blend
- √ 2 Tbsp. water

ALMOND ICING

- √ 2 cups powdered sugar

- √ 1 tsp. almond extract
- √ milk

EGG LAYER

- √ ½ cup coconut oil
- √ 1 cup of water
- √ 1 tsp. almond extract
- √ 1 cup flour blend
- √ 3 eggs

Directions:

Base Layer: Cut small pieces of butter into the flour mixture. Sprinkle water and combine. Press into an 8 × 8 pan.

Egg Layer: Melt butter, stir in flour and almond extract. Remove from heat. Put the eggs one at a time and mix

Spread over the base layer and bake at 350 degrees for 50–60 minutes or until topping is crisp and golden brown.

Top with icing and almonds.

Nutrition:

Calories: 231

Fat: 5g

Fiber: 3.8g

Carbs: 28.1g

Protein: 3.7g

4. Gluten-free Pancakes

Ingredients:

Pancake Mix:

- √ 6 cups rice flour
- √ 2 cups Cornstarch
- √ 4 tsp. salt

Dairy-free/ Vegan

Preparation Time: 15 minutes

Cooking Time: 15-20 minutes

Servings: 8

Difficulty: Easy

- √ 4 tsp. baking soda
- √ ¼ cup baking powder
- √ 4 tsp. xanthan gum
- √ ¾ cup of sugar

Directions:

Whisk a cup of pancake mix, mayonnaise about 2 tbsp, 1 cup water, and 1 egg. Pour batter in a skillet and cook on both sides.

Nutrition:

Calories: 201

Fat: 3.4g

Fiber: 8.5g

Carbs: 14.7g

Protein: 0.7g

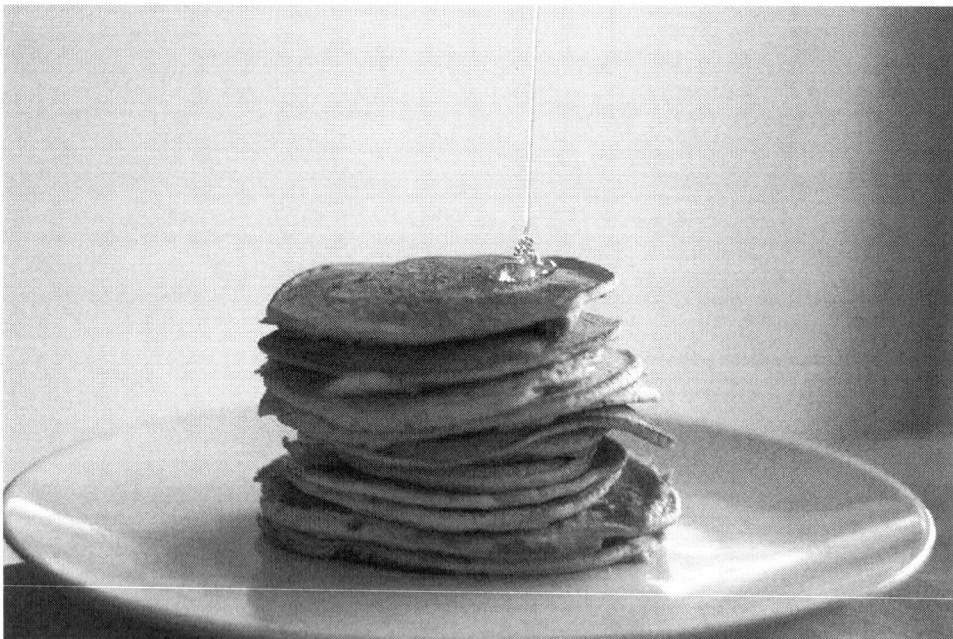

5. Breakfast Cheese Biscuits

Ingredients:

- √ ⅓ cup vegan butter
- √ 2 cups Gluten-Free *Pancake Mix*
- √ ⅔ cup almond milk
- √ 3 large eggs
- √ ⅓ cup grated dairy-free cheese

Dairy-free

Preparation Time: 15 minutes

Cooking Time: 15 minutes

Servings: 6

Difficulty: Easy

Directions: Oven: 400°F

Spray baking sheet with cooking spray.

Knead butter into the baking mix Add remaining ingredients and mix. Reserve some cheese for topping.

Making use of a large spoon, drop onto the sheet, and sprinkle with remaining cheese. Bake for 15 minutes until slightly brown.

Nutrition:

Calories: 181

Fat: 3.8g

Fiber: 2.8g

Carbs: 19.2g

Protein: 3.8 g

6. Baked Eggs in Squash

Ingredients:

- √ 4 acorn squash slices
- √ 1 tablespoon olive oil
- √ 4 eggs
- √ Pepper and salt

Dairy-free/ Vegetarian-friendly

Preparation Time: 15 minutes

Cooking Time: 20 minutes

Servings: 4

Difficulty: Easy

Toppings:

- √ 2 cups white mushrooms
- √ 2 tablespoons pumpkin seeds

- √ 1 tablespoon olive oil
- √ Pepper and salt
- √ parsley, to top
- √ avocado slices

Directions: Oven: 425°F

Brush all sides of each acorn squash slice with oil and bake them for 15 minutes. Spray the center of the squash slices with oil. Crack one piece of the egg to the center of each squash. Sprinkle with salt, and black pepper then bake for 6–10 minutes

Sauté the mushrooms and pumpkin seeds, about 6–8 minutes. Season.

Serve the baked eggs in squash topped with the mushrooms and pumpkin seeds, minced parsley, and avocado slices.

Nutrition:

Calories: 165

Fat: 4.3g

Fiber: 2.8g

Carbs: 9.9g

Protein: 10.7g

7. Breakfast Sweet Potato Sliders

Ingredients:

Dairy-free

- √ 6 sweet potato slices
- √ 2 teaspoons coconut oil
- √ ½ avocado smashed
- √ Pinch of salt
- √ 3 slices tomato
- √ 3 slices turkey meat

Preparation Time: 15 minutes

Cooking Time: 15 minutes

Servings: 3

Difficulty: Easy

Directions: Oven: 425°F

Brush all side of sweet potato slices in coconut oil and bake for 15–20 minutes, flipping halfway through.

In a bowl or container, combine the salt and avocado.

Sliders: Spread the avocado on a baked sweet potato slice, top with the tomato and turkey meat, then spread more avocado on the bottom of another baked sweet potato slice and place it on top.

Nutrition:

Calories: 265

Fat: 9.5g

Fiber: 3.9g

Carbs: 31.1g

Protein: 11g

8. Scotch Eggs

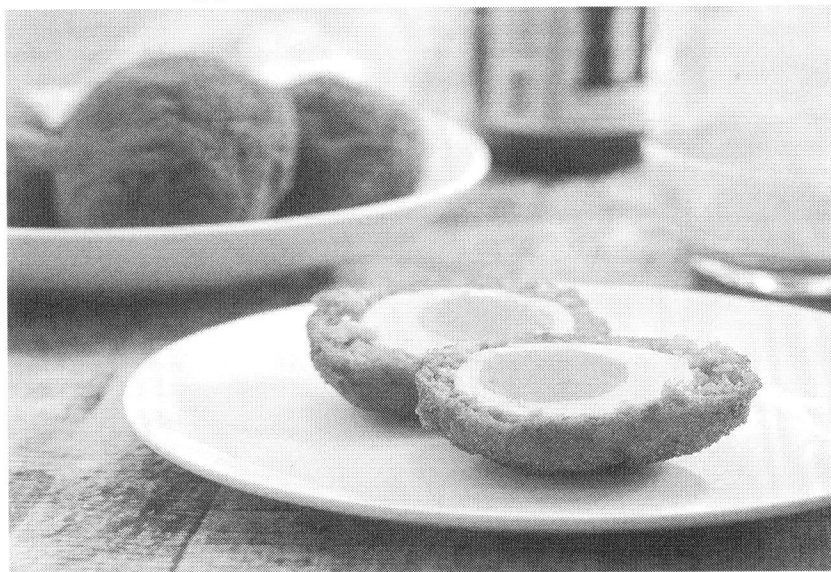

Ingredients:

√ 4 eggs

√ ½ pound ground beef

√ 1 teaspoon rosemary

√ ¼ teaspoon nutmeg

√ ½ teaspoon garlic powder

√ ½ teaspoon onion powder

√ Pepper and salt

Dairy-free/ Vegetarian-friendly

Preparation Time: 30 minutes

Cooking Time: 30 minutes

Servings: 2

Difficulty: Hard

√ ¼ teaspoon crushed red pepper

Almond Meal Crust:

√ 1 egg
√ ¼ cup almond milk
√ ⅓ cup almond meal
√ Salt

Directions: Oven: 425°F.

Boil your eggs anywhere from 9 minutes. After cooking, peel them

Combine the seasonings with the ground beef in a bowl. Separate the seasoned beef into four equal parts. In a separate bowl, the almond milk and egg must be combined. In another container or bowl, combine the salt and almond meal. Take the beef and shape into a patty then take the boiled egg and mold the beef around the egg, making sure no egg white is showing through.

Dip each covered egg in the egg wash; almond meal until completely covered.

Bake for 25–30 minutes or until the outer crust is browned and the beef is cooked through. Serve.

Nutrition:

Calories: 312

Fat: 15.9g

Fiber: 5.1g

Carbs: 31.7g

Protein: 3.5g

9. Skillet Breakfast

Ingredients:

√ 1 bell pepper, chopped
√ 1/2 onion, chopped
√ 6 button mushrooms, chopped
√ 1 clove garlic, minced
√ 3 tablespoons olive oil
√ 3 medium white potatoes, cooked and diced

Dairy-free/ Vegan

Preparation Time: 15 minutes

Cooking Time: 20 minutes

Servings: 4

Difficulty: Easy

√   1 tomato, chopped

Directions:

Saute pepper, onion, mushrooms, and garlic in olive oil until tender.

Put in the potatoes continue cooking until browned.

Add tomato and cook until mixture is heated through.

Nutrition:

Calories: 271

Fat: 10 g

Fiber: 2.5g

Carbs: 10.4g

Protein: 5.9 g

10. Crispy Potato Pancakes

Ingredients:

√   4 potatoesgrated
√   2 onions, minced
√   2 eggs
√   1/2 cup rice flour
√   Pepper and salt
√   2 cups olive oil

Dairy-free/ Vegan

Preparation Time: 20 minutes
Cooking Time: 20 minutes
Servings: 10
Difficulty: Easy

Garnish:

√   Applesauce, fruit preserves, salsa, or chutney

Directions:

In a container, mix all ingredients except oil and garnishes. Spoon in the potato cakes, pressing down to make a patty. Fry about 5 minutes per side. Serve with a garnish of choice.

Nutrition:

Calories: 219

Fat: 11.4g

Fiber: 4.9g

Carbs: 11.9g

Protein: 15.4g

11. Mushroom Scramble

Ingredients:

Vegetarian-friendly

- √ 4 egg whites
- √ 8 eggs
- √ 2 tablespoons almond milk
- √ 2 tablespoons Worcestershire sauce
- √ 2 cloves garlic, crushed
- √ 2 teaspoons olive oil
- √ 12 mushrooms
- √ 2 tablespoons parsley
- √ Pepper and salt

Preparation Time: 10 minutes

Cooking Time: 10 minutes

Servings: 4

Difficulty: Easy

Directions:

In a container, whisk together all the eggs, salt and pepper. Set aside.

In a heated saute pan, cook the remaining ingredients except the parsley. Add in the egg mix and scramble. Top with parsley and serve.

Nutrition:

Calories: 224

Fat: 12.5g

Fiber: 5.5g

Carbs: 19.5g

Protein: 14.5g

12. Waffles

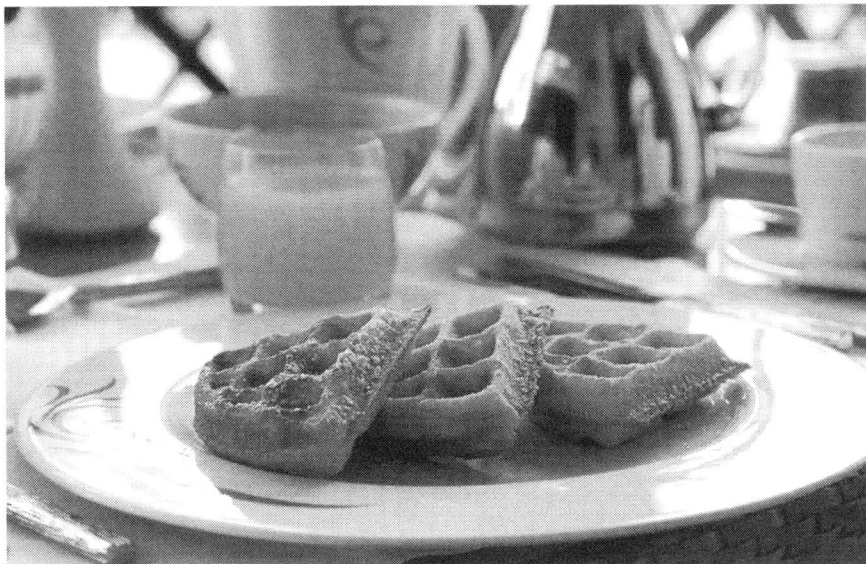

Ingredients:

- √ 1 cup Gluten-Free Flour
- √ 2 tsp baking powder
- √ ¼ tsp salt
- √ 1 tbsp sugar
- √ 2 eggs
- √ 1 cup milk
- √ 3 tbsp oil

Vegetarian-friendly

Preparation Time: 15 minutes

Cooking Time: 15 minutes

Servings: 6

Difficulty: Easy

Directions:

All of the ingredients must be combined in a container or bowl and whisk until smooth.

Heat waffle iron and pour batter. Waffles should be light golden brown when they are done.

Nutrition:

Calories: 201

Fat: 3.5g

Fiber: 2.1g

Carbs: 22.9g

Protein: 3.1g

13. Baked Tomato and Eggs

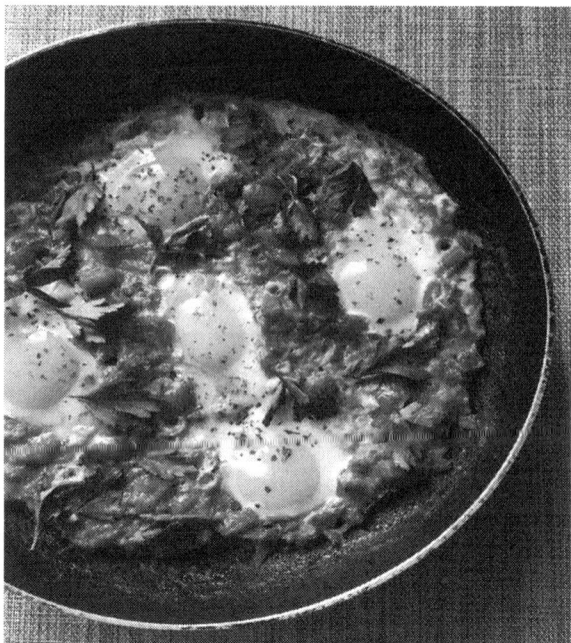

Ingredients:

- √ 1 tablespoon olive oil
- √ 1 red chili, finely chopped
- √ 2 chopped onions
- √ 1 sliced garlic clove
- √ 4 eggs
- √ 2 (400g) cans tomato
- √ Coriander leaves
- √ 1 teaspoon caster sugar

Dairy-free/ Vegetarian-friendly

Preparation Time: 15 minutes
Cooking Time: 18 minutes
Servings: 2
Difficulty: Medium

Directions:

Heat olive oil and saute onions, chili, coriander stalks, and garlic. Once soft, add in the sugar and tomatoes then bubble the mix for 8-10 minutes until thick. Crack in an egg into each. Cook until egg is set. Top coriander and serve with crusty bread.

Nutrition:

Calories: 171

Fat: 4.5g

Fiber: 4.1g

Carbs: 8.4g

Protein: 8.5g

14. Mini Quiche Bites

Ingredients:

Vegetarian-friendly

- √ 1 tablespoon olive oil
- √ ¼ cup diced onion
- √ 1 cup spinach leaves
- √ 1/2 cup mozzarella cheese
- √ ¼ cup milk
- √ Pepper and Salt
- √ 4 large eggs

Preparation Time: 15 minutes

Cooking Time: 20 minutes

Servings: 6

Difficulty: Easy

Directions: Oven: 350°F

Coat 6 muffin cups with cooking spray. In a heated skillet, saute onion and spinach until soft. Transfer spinach mixture to a small bowl. Cool for 3 minutes. Stir in cheese.

Combine milk and remaining ingredients, Stir in cheese mixture. Divide mixture into the muffin cups. Bake for 20 minutes.

Nutrition:

Calories: 150

Fat: 3.5g

Fiber: 4.1g

Carbs: 16.1g

Protein: 5.7g

15. Crepes with Blueberry and Coconut Cream

Ingredients:

Dairy-free/ Vegetarian-friendly

Crepe Batter:

- √ 1½ cups almond milk

Preparation Time: 15 minutes

Cooking Time: 20 minutes

- √ 2 eggs
- √ 1½ tablespoons honey
- √ 1 tablespoon coconut oil
- √ ¼ teaspoon salt
- √ 1 cup gluten-free flour

Blueberry Sauce:

- √ 1 cup blueberries
- √ 1 tablespoon lemon juice
- √ 1 tsp honey

Coconut Whipped Cream:

- √ 1 can coconut milk (placed in the refrigerator for at least 12 hours)
- √ 2 teaspoons honey
- √ ¼ teaspoon cinnamon

Directions:

In a bowl or container, mix all crepe batter ingredients until smooth.Chill in the refrigerator.

For the coconut cream, using an electric hand mixer, blend all ingredients until peaks begin to form

Blueberry sauce: Put all ingredients in a food processor and process until the sauce is completely smooth.

To make the crepes, heat a small nonstick skillet. The pan must be greased with a nonstick cooking spray and scoop the batter to the center of the pan. To spread the batter out thin and evenly, swirl the pan. Cook the crepe for 30 seconds, then gently flip it and cook the other side for 10–15 seconds.

Serve the crepes rolled, topped with the blueberry sauce, and a dollop of the cinnamon-coconut whipped cream.

Nutrition:

Calories: 276

Fat: 5.4g

Fiber: 9.5g

Carbs:28.5g

Protein: 3.7g

16. Egg and Hash Brown Cups

Ingredients:

- √ 3 cups grated potatoes
- √ ½ teaspoon salt
- √ 5 eggs
- √ ½ teaspoon thyme
- √ ¼ teaspoon red pepper
- √ Black pepper
- √ Serve with ketchup

Dairy-free/ Vegetarian-friendly

Preparation Time: 15 minutes

Cooking Time: 30 minutes

Servings: 5

Difficulty: Medium

Directions: Oven: 425°F

Grease muffin pans then place the grated potatoes in the muffin slots and gently press the potatoes down, creating a cup. Season with salt and bake for 15 minutes.

Crack each egg into the hash brown cups then top with remaining seasonings. Bake for 15 minutes.

Serve with Ketchup.

Nutrition:

Calories: 134

Fat: 4.2g

Fiber: 1.5g

Carbs: 11.7g

Protein: 5.7g

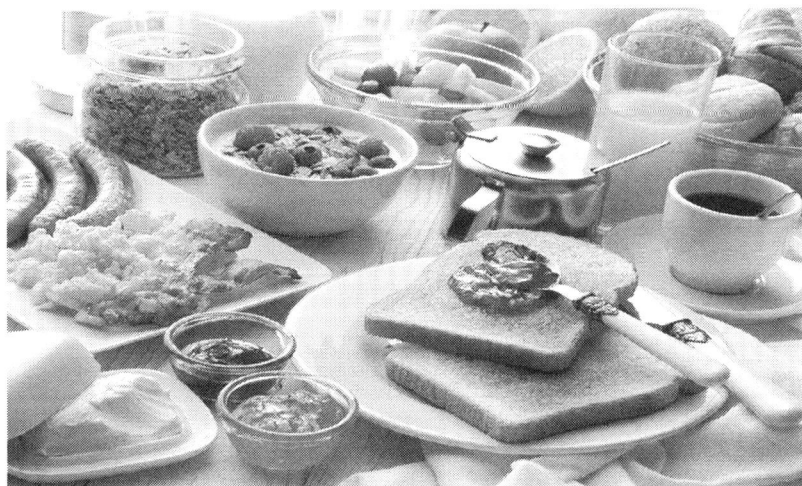

Chapter 3. <u>CAKES AND CHEESECAKES</u>

17. Chocolate Cake

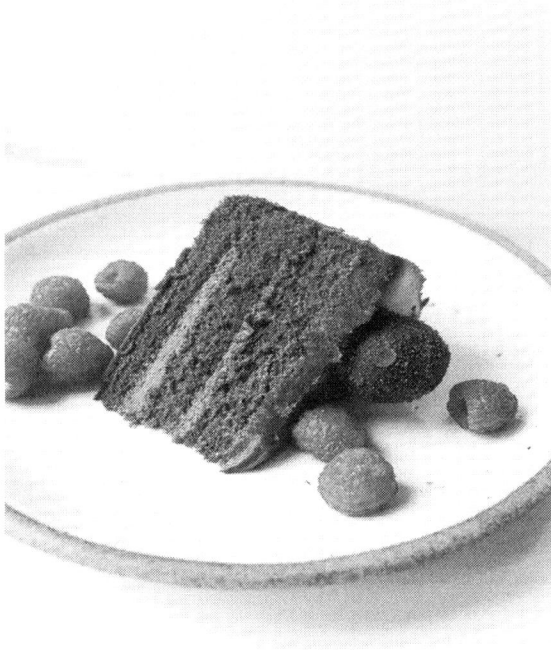

Ingredients:

- √ ½ cup rice flour
- √ ¼ cup sorghum flour
- √ ¼ cup almond flour
- √ ½ cup tapioca starch
- √ ¼ cup potato starch
- √ ½ tsp. gelatin
- √ ¼ tsp. salt
- √ 1½ tsp. baking powder
- √ 1 tsp. baking soda
- √ 1½ cups sugar
- √ 4 eggs
- √ 2 tsp. vanilla extract
- √ 1 cup sour cream
- √ 1 cup of coconut oil

Dairy-free/ Vegetarian-friendly

Preparation Time: 20 minutes

Cooking Time: 25 minutes

Servings: 8

Difficulty: Medium

- √ ¾ cup chocolate chips
- √ ½ cup cacao powder

Directions: Oven: 350°F

Cream together sugar, eggs, and vanilla. After it is well combined, add the sour cream. Add the dry ingredients to the wet mixture. Set aside

In a heated saucepan, the butter, coconut oil & chocolate chips must be melted. Whisk in cocoa powder. Add the chocolate mixture to the other bowl. Pour cake batter into two 9" cake pans. Bake for 25–27 minutes.

Nutrition:

Calories: 209

Fat: 11.2g

Fiber: 4.1g

Carbs: 23.5g

Protein: 4.7g

18. Tres Leches

Ingredients:

Vegetarian-friendly

- √ ⅓ cup sorghum flour
- √ ⅓ cup coconut flour
- √ 1 cup white rice flour
- √ ½ cup tapioca starch
- √ ½ cup potato starch
- √ ⅓ cup cornstarch
- √ 1 tsp. gelatin
- √ 1 Tbsp. baking powder
- √ 1 tsp. Salt
- √ 2 cups of sugar
- √ ½ cup vegan butter or shortening
- √ ½ cup coconut oil softened
- √ 1 tsp. vanilla extract

Preparation Time: 30 minutes

Cooking Time: 45 minutes

Servings: 6

Difficulty: Medium

- √   1½ cups almond milk
- √   6 eggs

TRES LECHES SYRUP

- √   2 (14-oz.) cans coconut milk
- √   1 cup coconut cream
- √   1 cup heavy whipping cream

TOPPING

- √   1 cup heavy whipping cream
- √   ⅓ cup powdered sugar
- √   Cinnamon and nutmeg

Directions: Oven: 350°F

Cream together sugar, butter, coconut oil, and vanilla. Add the eggs one at a time then mix in in the milk.

In a bowl, the remaining dry ingredients must be combined. Combine the two mixtures. Make sure Pour batter to a 9 × 13 baking pan and bake for approximately 45 minutes.

Tres Leches Syrup: Whisk all listed ingredients.

Use a wooden skewer to poke 2–3 dozen holes throughout the cake. Pour the syrup over the cake, wait to let the syrup soak in then pour on more. Put some cover and chill for 8 hours.

Add the powdered sugar to the remaining cup of cream and whip lightly. Spread the whipping cream over the top and sprinkle with a little nutmeg and cinnamon.

Nutrition:

Calories: 211

Fat: 12.1g

Fiber: 5.5g

Carbs: 24.5g

Protein: 7.4 g

19. Almond Crust Cheesecake

Ingredients:

Vegetarian-friendly

Crust:

- √ ½ cup slivered almonds
- √ 1 cup almond meal
- √ ¼ cup of sugar
- √ ¼ tsp. salt
- √ ¼ tsp. cinnamon
- √ ¼ tsp. baking soda
- √ ¼ cup coconut oil

Cheesecake:

- √ 19 oz. cream cheese (vegetarian)
- √ 1 cup of sugar
- √ ½ tsp. vanilla extract
- √ 3 large eggs

Preparation Time: 35 minutes

Cooking Time: 10 minutes

Servings: 8

Difficulty: Medium

Directions:

Oven: 350°F

Crush slivered almonds and combine them in a large bowl with remaining crust ingredients. Press into a parchment paper-lined pie pan. Bake for 10 minutes. Set aside to cool.

Turn oven down to 300°F. In a bowl or container, beat together cheesecake ingredients on high, about 3 minutes. Pour into prepared crust and bake at for 1 hour.

Let cool slightly before chilling in the refrigerator.

Nutrition:

Calories: 298

Fat: 15.4g

Fiber: 9.4g

Carbs: 33.1g

Protein: 2.4 g

20. Coffee Chocolate Bundt Cake

Ingredients:

Dairy-free/ Vegetarian

- √ ⅔ cup coconut oil
- √ 1½ cups brown sugar
- √ 2 large eggs
- √ 2 teaspoons vanilla extract
- √ ½ cup almond milk
- √ 2⅔ cups Gluten-Free Flour
- √ ⅔ cup cocoa powder
- √ 1½ teaspoons xanthan gum
- √ 1 teaspoon baking soda
- √ ½ teaspoon salt
- √ 1 cup hot brewed coffee

Preparation Time: 15 minutes

Cooking Time: 55 minutes

Servings: 12

Difficulty: Medium

Directions:

Oven: 350°F

Grease Bundt pan.

In a container, beat the sugar and butter for 2 minutes. Beat in the eggs, vanilla, and milk until well blended.

In another bowl, whisk the dry ingredients together. Alternately put in the dry ingredients and the warm coffee until the batter is mixed. Spread the batter evenly in the pan.

Bake the bundt cake for about 50 to 55 minutes.

Nutrition:

Calories: 298

Fat: 15.1g

Fiber: 9.4g

Carbs: 31.2g

Protein: 4.5g

21. Butter Bundt Cake

Ingredients:

- √ ½ cup vegan butter or coconut oil
- √ 1¼ cups sugar
- √ 2 large eggs
- √ 2 cups Gluten-Free Flour
- √ 2 teaspoons baking powder
- √ 1 teaspoon xanthan gum
- √ ½ teaspoon salt
- √ ⅛ teaspoon baking soda
- √ ¼ cup water
- √ 1 tablespoon lemon zest
- √ 2 teaspoons vanilla extract

Dairy-free / Vegetarian-Friendly

Preparation Time: 15 minutes

Cooking Time: 55 minutes

Servings: 12

Difficulty: Medium

Directions:

Oven: 350°F

Grease Bundt pan.

In a bowl or container, cream the sugar and butter then continue by adding in the eggs one by one.

In another container or bowl, whisk together the all dry ingredients. Mix the water, lemon zest and vanilla. Mix the egg and flour mixture gradually. Spread the batter evenly in the pan.

Let it bake until the top is golden brown, 50 to 55 minutes.

Nutrition:

Calories: 287

Fat: 15.4g

Fiber: 7.2g

Carbs: 33.7g

Protein: 4.1g

22. New York Cheesecake

Ingredients:

Vegetarian-friendly

FOR THE CRUST

- √ ¼ teaspoon coconut oil or avocado oil
- √ 2 cups gluten-free graham cracker crumbs
- √ ⅓ cup brown sugar
- √ 8 tablespoons melted butter

Preparation Time: 25 minutes

Cooking Time: 1 hr. and 15 minutes
Servings: 12
Difficulty: Hard

FOR THE FILLING

- √ 5 (8-ounce) packages cream cheese
- √ 5 large eggs
- √ 1 cup granulated sugar
- √ 1 cup sour cream
- √ ¼ cup almond flour
- √ 1 tablespoon vanilla extract

Directions: Oven: 325°F A 9-inch springform pan must be greased.

In a container, stir together the graham crumbs and sugar then Drizzle the butter over it then mix again.

Transfer the crust to the springform pan and press firmly into place across the bottom and ½ inch up the sides of the pan. Bake for 10 minutes.

FILLING:

Put cream cheese in stand mixer's bowl and beat until smooth. Add in the eggs one by one. Then the sugar sour cream, flour and vanilla. Beat until fully incorporated.

CHEESECAKE:

Spoon the filling into the crust.

Bake for 1 hour and 10 minutes.

Nutrition:

Calories: 301

Fat: 11.5g

Fiber: 4.9g

Carbs: 33.7g

Protein: 6.4 g

23. Blueberry Coffee Cake

Ingredients:

Vegetarian-friendly

FOR THE BATTER

Preparation Time: 15 minutes

- √ ¼ teaspoon coconut oil
- √ 1½ cups gluten-free flour
- √ ½ cup granulated sugar
- √ 2 large eggs
- √ ½ cup coconut milk
- √ 2 tablespoons sunflower oil
- √ Juice of 1 lemon
- √ 1 cup blueberries

Cooking Time: 25 minutes
Servings: 8
Difficulty: Medium

FOR THE STREUSEL

- √ ⅔ cup almond flour
- √ ½ cup granulated sugar
- √ 1½ teaspoons cinnamon
- √ ¼ cup dairy-free butter
- √ Lemon Zest

Directions: Oven: 325°F. The pan must then be greased with the oil.

Batter:

Stir together all the batter ingredients. Gently fold in the blueberries then pour into the baking pan.

Streusel:

In a bowl or container all streusel ingredients.

Top the batter with the streusel, gently pressing it into the batter.

Bake for 20 to 25 minutes.

Nutrition:

Calories: 287

Fat: 12.5g

Fiber: 3.9g

Carbs: 31.9g

Protein: 4.9g

24. Triple Berry Cheesecake

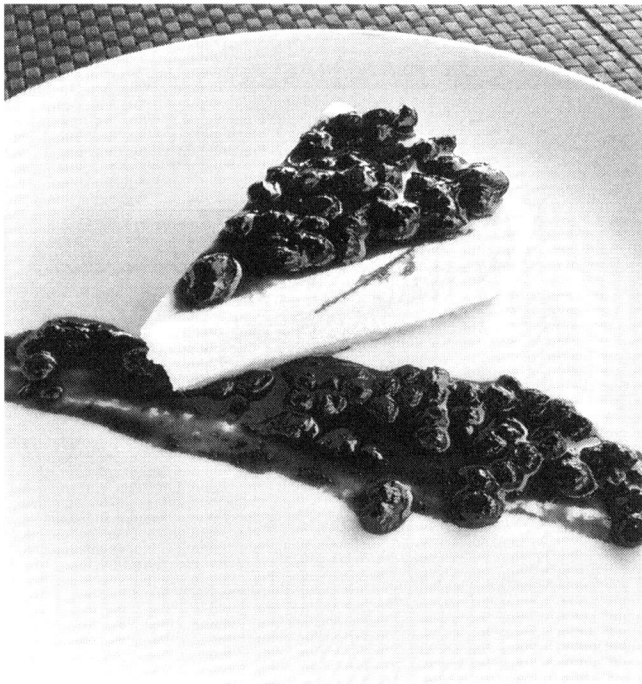

Ingredients:

CRUST

- √ 6 tablespoons nondairy butter
- √ 1 cup gluten-free rolled oats
- √ 1 cup tapioca flour
- √ 1 cup dry unsweetened coconut
- √ 6 tablespoons maple syrup
- √ Salt

Dairy-free/ Vegetarian-friendly

Preparation Time: 40 minutes

Cooking Time: 10 minutes

Servings: 12

Difficulty: Hard

GELATIN MIX:

- √ ½ cup of water
- √ 1½ teaspoons agar-agar

FILLING AND TOPPING

- √ ½ teaspoon salt
- √ 16 ounces non-dairy cream cheese
- √ ½ cup canned coconut milk
- √ 1 tablespoon nutritional yeast
- √ 1 teaspoon vanilla extract
- √ ⅔ cup honey
- √ Topping:
- √ 1½ cups mixed berries

Directions:

Oven: 350°F

In a food processor, pulse all crust ingredients. Press the mixture onto the base of the springform pan. Let the cheesecake bake for 10 minutes while preparing the filling. Set aside.

FILLING:

In a heated saucepan, combine the salt and water and sprinkle with gelatin then bring to a boil.

In a container, beat all filling ingredients. Incorporate the gelatin mixture then blend well. Pour this to the crust and until firm.

Garnish with berries and drizzled with honey.

Nutrition:

Calories: 314

Fat: 7.4g

Fiber: 8.5g

Carbs: 34.1g

Protein: 5.4 g

25. Butter Pound Cake

Ingredients:

Dry Ingredients:

- √ 2 cups gluten-free flour
- √ ¼ cup arrowroot
- √ 1 tablespoon baking powder
- √ 1 teaspoon xanthan gum
- √ ¼ teaspoon salt

Wet Ingredients:

- √ 1 cup honey
- √ 1 cup vegan butter
- √ 4 large eggs
- √ 1 teaspoon vinegar
- √ 1 teaspoon vanilla extract
- √ ¼ cup sour cream

Topping:

- √ Confectioners' sugar

Vegetarian-friendly

Preparation Time: 15 minutes

Cooking Time: 60 minutes

Servings: 12

Difficulty: Medium

Directions: Oven: 350°F

In a container, all dry ingredients must be combined.

In another container, beat the honey and butter together until fluffy. Beat in remaining wet ingredients. Pour into the 9" pan. Bake it for about an hour. Dust with confectioners' sugar before serving.

Nutrition:

Calories: 298

Fat: 16.4g

Fiber: 4.4g

Carbs: 31.7g

Protein: 3.4g

26. Zucchini Bundt Cake

Ingredients:

Dry Ingredients:

- √ 3 cups gluten-free flour
- √ 1 tablespoon baking powder
- √ 1½ teaspoons cinnamon
- √ 1½ teaspoons xanthan gum
- √ 1 teaspoon baking soda
- √ 1 teaspoon salt

Wet Ingredients:

- √ 3 large eggs
- √ 1 cup coconut sugar
- √ 1 cup avocado oil
- √ ½ cup maple syrup
- √ 1 tablespoon vanilla extract
- √ 2 cups grated zucchini, with water squeezed out
- √ ½ cup chopped walnuts

Dairy-free/ Vegetarian-friendly

Preparation Time: 15 minutes

Cooking Time: 55 minutes

Servings: 12

Difficulty: Medium

Directions: Oven: 350°F

Coat a 9-inch Bundt pan with cooking spray and flour.

In a container, all dry ingredients must be combined

In another container, beat the eggs until light and creamy. Beat in the remaining dry ingredients. Fold in the walnuts. Pour into the prepared pan.

Bake the Bundt cake for around 50 to 55 minutes.

Nutrition:

Calories: 287

Fat: 11.5g

Fiber: 4.9g

Carbs: 33.4g

Protein: 5.4 g

27. No-Bake Cherry Cheesecake

Ingredients:

Crust:

- √ 2 cups gluten-free pretzels
- √ 1 tablespoon brown sugar
- √ ½ cup melted vegan butter/ coconut oil

Filling:

- √ 2 packages cream cheese
- √ 1 cup sour cream
- √ 1 cup powdered sugar
- √ 1 teaspoon vanilla extract

Topping:

- √ 1 can gluten-free cherry pie filling

Vegetarian-friendly

Preparation Time: 15 minutes

Cooking Time: 25 minutes

Servings: 9

Difficulty: Easy

Directions:

Pulse all the crust mixture then press into an 8-by-8-inch baking dish.

In a container, whip all filling ingredients. Spread this mixture over the crust. Let it freeze for 15 more minutes. Spread the cherry pie filling over the cheesecake.

Nutrition:

Calories: 288

Fat: 15g

Fiber: 4.9g

Carbs: 31.9g

Protein: 7.6 g

28. Spiced Cake

Ingredients:

Dry:

- √ 1¼ cups Gluten-Free Flour

Vegetarian-friendly

Preparation Time: 15 minutes

Cooking Time: 30 minutes

- √ 2 tsp baking powder
- √ ½ tsp salt
- √ 1 tsp cinnamon
- √ ¼ tsp ground nutmeg and cloves
- √ ½ cup brown sugar
- √ ¼ cup of sugar

Wet:

- √ ¼ cup vegan butter/coconut oil
- √ ¾ cup almond milk
- √ 1 tsp vanilla
- √ 2 eggs

Servings: 8
Difficulty: Medium

Directions: Oven: 350°F

In a container, all wet ingredients must be combined.

In another container, combine all dry ingredients. Mix the two mixture together.

Pour batter into a greased and floured 9" round baking pan. Let it bake for about 30 minutes.

Nutrition:

Calories: 222

Fat: 14.1g

Fiber: 3.9g

Carbs: 31.9g

Protein: 1.4g

29. Apple Upside Down Cake

Ingredients:

CARAMEL SAUCE

- √ ¾ cup of brown sugar
- √ ½ cup coconut milk
- √ ½ teaspoon vanilla extract
- √ salt

Dairy-free/ Vegan

Preparation Time: 25 minutes

Cooking Time: 55 minutes

Servings: 10

Difficulty: Hard

CAKE

- √ 2 flax eggs (4 tablespoons water +2 tablespoons ground flaxseed)
- √ ¾ cup coconut milk
- √ 1 teaspoon apple cider vinegar
- √ 1¼ cups rice flour
- √ 1¼ cups almond flour
- √ ¾ cup of brown sugar
- √ 1 tablespoon apple pie spice
- √ 1½ teaspoons baking powder
- √ ½ teaspoon baking soda
- √ ¼ teaspoon of salt
- √ ¾ cup applesauce
- √ ¼ cup maple syrup
- √ 1 teaspoon vanilla extract
- √ 2 tablespoons coconut oil
- √ 2 cups thinly sliced apple

Directions: Oven: 350°F

Caramel sauce: In a heated saucepan, combine all ingredients and cook on low heat for 10 minutes.

Spray an 8-inch round spring-form cake pan with cooking spray. In a bowl or container, combine all cake dry ingredients. Do the same with the wet ingredients except the apple slices. Combine both mixtures. Pour the caramel sauce in the bottom of the prepared cake pan. Layer in the sliced apple. Pour the batter on top of the apples. Let it bake for about 55 minutes.

Nutrition:

Calories: 243

Fat: 11.5g

Fiber: 4.1g

Carbs: 32.1g

Protein: 2.4g

30. Lemon Cheesecake

Ingredients:

CRUST:

- √ 3 cups gluten-free gingersnap cookie crumbs
- √ ¾ cup coconut oil
- √ 3 Tbsp. sugar

LEMON CREAM FILLING:

- √ 4 (8-oz.) pkgs. cream cheese
- √ 4 eggs
- √ 2 cups sugar
- √ ½ cup lemon juice
- √ 16 oz. sour cream
- √ 3 Tbsp. Powdered sugar
- √ ½ tsp. vanilla

GINGERSNAP CRUMBS:

- √ ¼ cup almond flour
- √ ¼ cup brown rice flour
- √ ¼ cup sorghum flour
- √ ¼ cup coconut flour
- √ ⅓ cup tapioca starch
- √ ½ cup potato starch
- √ ¾ tsp. gelatin powder
- √ 1 tsp. Baking powder
- √ ¼ tsp. Salt
- √ ¾ cup sugar
- √ ¼ cup molasses
- √ 4 Tbsp coconut oil
- √ 1 egg
- √ 2 tsp. cinnamon
- √ 2 tsp. ground ginger

Vegetarian-friendly

Preparation Time: 40 minutes

Cooking Time: 1 hr. 15 minutes
Servings: 8
Difficulty: Medium

Directions: Oven: 350°F

Preheat oven to 350 degrees. Combine all crust ingredients and press into the bottom and up sides of a springform pan.

Using a stand mixer with the whisk, whip all filling ingredients. Pour filling into crust. Bake for approximately 45 minutes.

Whip sour cream, powdered sugar, and vanilla together. Spread on the top of the cheesecake and return to the oven. Bake for an additional 10 minutes. Garnish with whipped cream and lemon slices.

Nutrition:

Calories: 243

Fat: 12.6g

Fiber: 9.5g

Carbs: 29.7g

Protein: 5.7g

31. Apple Bundt Cake

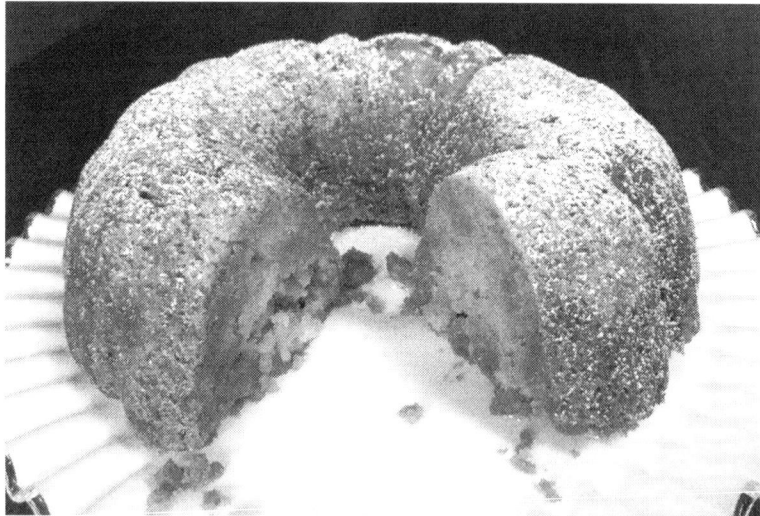

Ingredients:

CAKE

√ 1 cup almond milk

√ 1 tablespoon white vinegar

Dairy-free/Vegetarian-friendly

Preparation Time: 20 minutes

Cooking Time: 1 hr. and 10 minutes

Servings: 10

- √ 1 cup coconut oil
- √ 2 cups granulated sugar
- √ 4 eggs
- √ 1 tablespoon vanilla extract
- √ 3 cups gluten-free flour
- √ 1 teaspoon baking powder
- √ ½ teaspoon baking soda
- √ 1 tablespoon cinnamon
- √ 3 cups apples
- √ 1 cup pecans

Difficulty: Medium

GLAZE

- √ ⅓ cup coconut oil
- √ ¾ cup brown sugar
- √ 2 tablespoons water
- √ 2 teaspoons vanilla extract
- √ ¼ teaspoon cinnamon

Directions: Oven: 325°F

The Bundt pan must be sprayed with nonstick spray. Put in the vinegar and milk to a small bowl and allow to sit for 5 minutes to make buttermilk.

In a bowl or container, combine both dry and wet ingredients. Stir in apples and pecans. The batter must be poured in the Bundt pan and let the cake bake for 70 minutes.

Mix all the listed ingredients for the glaze in a medium-heated saucepan. Poke holes all over warm cake with a knife and pour glaze over cake while still in the pan.

Nutrition:

Calories: 281

Fat: 10.4g

Fiber: 6.4g

Carbs: 29.7g

Protein: 4.3g

32. Chocolate Cherry Cheesecake

Ingredients:

Dairy-free/ Vegetarian-friendly

CRUST:

- √ 1¼ cups almond flour
- √ ¼ cup of coconut sugar
- √ 2 tablespoons arrowroot starch
- √ 2 tablespoons cocoa powder
- √ ⅓ cup coconut oil

Preparation Time: 40 minutes

Cooking Time: 50 minutes

Servings: 12

Difficulty: Hard

FILLING:

- √ ½ cup chocolate chips
- √ 3 tablespoons coconut oil
- √ 1½ cups raw cashews, soaked in water overnight, drained and rinsed
- √ 1 (8-ounce) package vegan cheese
- √ ½ cup coconut milk
- √ ½ cup maple syrup
- √ ½ cup coconut cream
- √ 3 tablespoons cocoa powder
- √ 2 tablespoons arrowroot starch
- √ 1 teaspoon vanilla extract
- √ ¼ teaspoon salt

CHERRY TOPPING:

- √ 3 tablespoons coconut oil
- √ 2 cups cherries
- √ ⅓ cup white sugar
- √ 1 teaspoon vanilla extract
- √ 2 tablespoons arrowroot starch

Directions: Oven: 350°F

Spray an 8-inch round springform cake pan with nonstick spray.

Combine all the crust ingredients and in the bottom of the prepared cake pan, press it firmly.

Let it bake for 10 minutes, and after baking, set it aside.

To make the filling, in a small saucepan, mix the dairy-free chocolate chips and coconut oil. Cook over medium heat until melted. Remove from the heat and set aside.

In a high-speed blender, mix remaining filling ingredients and blend until everything is smooth. The melted chocolate will then be incorporated and blended.

Pour the filling into the cake pan with the crust. Let it bake for about 50 minutes

Make the topping by combining all in a saucepan until thickened. Pour on top of the chilled cheesecake

Nutrition:

Calories: 298

Fat: 15g

Fiber: 4.6g

Carbs: 33.4g

Protein: 8.4 g

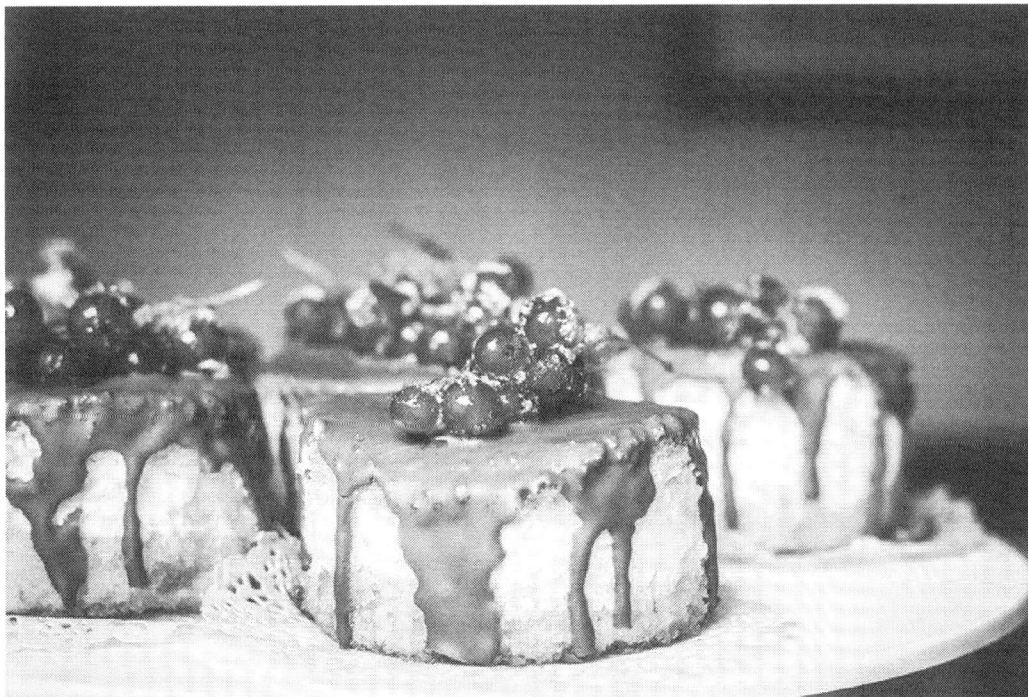

Chapter 4. <u>PIES, TARTS AND CRUMBLES</u>

33. Basic Gluten-Free Pie Crust

Dry Ingredients:

Dairy-free

- √ 1/2 cup Tapioca starch
- √ ½ cup coconut flour
- √ 1 cup almond flour
- √ 1 teaspoon salt
- √ 1 teaspoon xantham fum
- √ Other ingredients:
- √ 2/3 cup shortening, chilled
- √ 5 tablespoons cold water

Preparation Time: 35 minutes

Cooking Time: 0 minutes

Servings: 1 pie crust

Difficulty: Easy

Directions:

In a container, mix all dry ingredients; next, cut in the cold shortening by making use of a pastry blender. Then, add in water until it becomes one dough. Now, you can use it or chill it for further use.

Nutrition:

Calories: 165

Fat: 3.1g

Fiber: 1.5g

Carbs: 10.7g

Protein: 1.2 g

34. Key Lime Pie

Ingredients:

Dairy-free/ Vegetarian-friendly

- √ 1 recipe gluten-free pie crust

Filling:

- √ 5 ripe avocados
- √ 1 cup confectioners' sugar
- √ 1/2 cup lime juice

Preparation Time: 25 minutes

Cooking Time: 15 minutes

Servings: 8

Difficulty: Medium

- √ 1/3 cup lime zest
- √ 1/4 cup coconut oil
- √ 1 teaspoon vanilla extract
- √ 1/4 teaspoon salt

Directions: Oven: 350°F

Bake gluten-free pie crust for 15 minutes. Set aside and cool down.

In a blender add all filling ingredients and blend until pureed.

Pour the mixture into the pie crust. Cover the pie with plastic wrap then chill the pie until set.

Nutrition:

Calories: 175

Fat: 3.9g

Fiber: 2.1g

Carbs: 19.5g

Protein: 3.7g

35. Plum Tart

Ingredients:

- √ 1 recipe gluten-free pie crust, not rolled out

Filling:

- √ 1 1/2 pounds red plums
- √ 3/4 cup granulated sugar
- √ 1 tablespoon cornstarch

Dairy-free/ Vegetarian-friendly

Preparation Time: 30 minutes

Cooking Time: 40 minutes

Servings: 8

Difficulty: Easy

Directions: Oven: 400°F

Roll out the chilled pie crust, making the size bigger than the diameter of the pie pan then press the crust into a 9-inch tart pan. Trim the edges of the pie crust to fit the pan, then prick the crust all over with a fork. Let it bake for 12 minutes.

While waiting, combine filling ingredients in a heated sauté pan and cook for 10 minutes. Pour the plum mixture into the pie crust and return to the oven for 30 minutes.

Nutrition:

Calories: 192

Fat: 6.5g

Fiber: 2.5g

Carbs: 19.7g

Protein: 3.7g

36. Sweet Strawberry Tarts

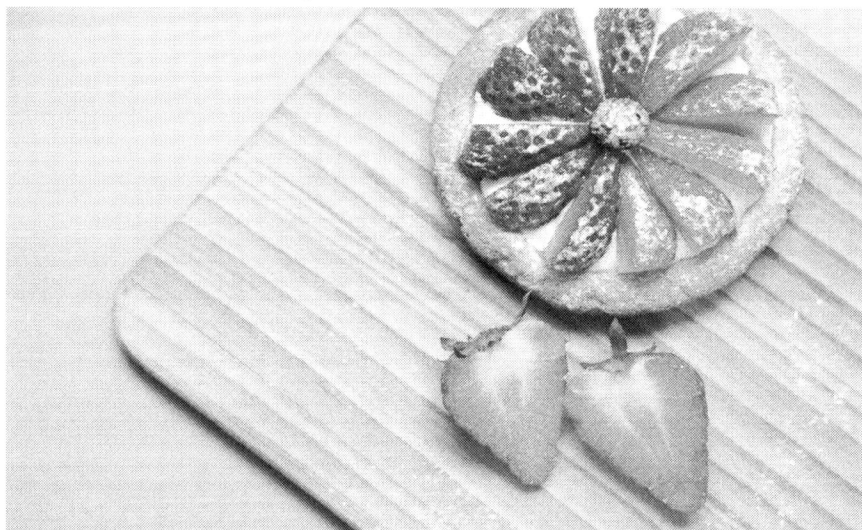

Ingredients:

Crust:

- √ ½ cup unsalted butter
- √ ¼ cup of sugar
- √ ¾ cup almond flour
- √ 1 tsp. vanilla extract

Filling:

- √ 2 ½ cups strawberries
- √ Lime zest
- √ ⅔ cup lime juice
- √ 1 cup of sugar

Dairy-free

Preparation Time: 40 minutes

Cooking Time: 35 minutes

Servings: 12

Difficulty: Medium

- √ 3 egg whites
- √ 1 egg
- √ ½ cup tapioca starch
- √ ⅛ tsp. salt

Directions: Oven: 375°F

Crust:

Mix all crust ingredients. The dough must be spread evenly into the bottom of the an 8 x 8 baking dish and bake for 20 minutes.

Filling:

Blend strawberries until smooth. Pour into a fine sieve to remove seeds and skin then place into a bowl. Add remaining ingredients and stir until combined. The mixture will be poured over the crust and bake for 35 minutes.

Top with strawberries and whipped cream when serving.

Nutrition:

Calories: 175

Fat: 4.5g

Fiber: 3.5g

Carbs: 17g

Protein: 1.1g

37. Raspberry-Peach Crumble

Ingredients:

FILLING:

Vegetarian-friendly/ Dairy Free

Preparation Time: 30 minutes

- √ 1/4 cup apple juice
- √ 1/4 teaspoon agar-agar
- √ 1 tablespoon honey
- √ 1 teaspoon vanilla
- √ 1/8 teaspoon cinnamon
- √ 4 ripe peaches, sliced

Cooking Time: 20 minutes

Servings: 4

Difficulty: Medium

√   1 cup raspberries

TOPPING:

√   1 cup almond flour
√   1/3 cup almonds
√   3 tablespoons coconut oil
√   1 tablespoon honey
√   1/8 teaspoon cinnamon
√   Salt

Directions: Oven: 350°F

In a bowl or container, add juice and sprinkle agar-agar over the top. For 5 minutes, let it sit to soften. Then whisk in the honey, vanilla, and cinnamon.

Add the peach slices and raspberries to the honey mixture and toss to coat thoroughly. Transfer to an 8" × 8" baking dish.

Topping:

In a bowl or container, combine the topping ingredients. Put the topping evenly over the peaches and raspberries. Let it bake for about 20 minutes.

Nutrition:

Calories: 174

Fat: 3.5g

Fiber: 2.1g

Carbs: 19.7g

Protein: 4.7g

38. Southern Sweet Potato Pie

Ingredients:

√   1 Gluten-Free Pie Crust

Filling:

√   2 cups sweet potato purée

Dairy-free/ Vegan

Preparation Time: 35 minutes

Cooking Time: 55 minutes

Servings: 8

- √ 1⁄2 cup maple syrup
- √ 1⁄2 teaspoon nutmeg
- √ 1⁄4 teaspoon ginger
- √ 1 teaspoon vanilla extract

Difficulty: Medium

Other ingredient:

- √ 2 tablespoons flaxseed meal + 4 tablespoons water OR 2 large eggs

Directions:

Oven: 425°F

Prebake pie crust for 5 minutes. In a bowl or container, combine filling ingredients.

In another container, combine flaxseed and water. Let sit for 3–4 minutes.

Mix flaxseed mixture into sweet potato mixture.

Pour filling into pie crust. Bake for 15 minutes.

The heat will then be lowered to 350°F and bake for another 40 minutes.

Nutrition:

Calories: 198

Fat: 11.5g

Fiber: 3.4g

Carbs: 29.7g

Protein: 2.4g

39. Strawberry Crumble

Ingredients:

- √ ¼ teaspoon coconut oil
- √ 6 cups strawberries
- √ ¼ cup of sugar
- √ ½ cup almond flour

Dairy-free/ Vegetarian-friendly

Preparation Time: 15 minutes

Cooking Time: 45 minutes

Servings: 8

Difficulty: Easy

Crumble:

- √ 1 cup gluten-free oats
- √ ½ cup brown sugar
- √ ¼ teaspoon salt
- √ ¼ cup vegan butter

Directions: Oven: 350°F

Place the strawberries in the pie plate and sprinkle with the sugar and 3 tablespoons of flour. Stir.

Place all crumble ingredients in a food processor. Pulse until the mixture resembles coarse crumbs. Spread the topping evenly over the strawberries. Let the crumble bake for 45 minutes.

Nutrition:

Calories: 215

Fat: 11.5g

Fiber: 4.2g

Carbs: 32.7g

Protein: 1.9g

40. Pecan Pie

Ingredients:

Crust:

- √ 1½ cups almond meal
- √ 6 tablespoons coconut oil
- √ 1½ cups cashews
- √ 1 large egg
- √ 1 large egg white
- √ 1 teaspoon vanilla extract
- √ 1 tablespoon coconut sugar

Filling:

- √ 3 tablespoons non-dairy butter
- √ ¾ cup corn syrup

Dairy-free

Preparation Time: 15 minutes

Cooking Time: 50 minutes

Servings: 8

Difficulty: Hard

- √ 3 large eggs
- √ ¼ cup of coconut sugar
- √ 2 teaspoons vanilla extract
- √ 1 teaspoon orange zest
- √ ¼ teaspoon salt

Other ingredients:

- √ 2 cups pecan halves

Directions: Oven: 350°F

Combine all crust ingredients in the food processor.

Press the crust into the pie pan then poke holes in the crust using a fork. Bake for 10 minutes.

Filling:

In a heated saucepan, melt the butter. Add remaining ingredients. Bring to a boil, whisking constantly. On the bottom of the pie crust, lay the pecans in a pattern. Pour the egg mixture over the pecans. Place the pie back in the oven and continue baking for 40 minutes.

Nutrition:

Calories: 276

Fat: 15g

Fiber: 6.5g

Carbs: 33.1g

Protein: 4.2g

41. Cottage Pie

Ingredients:

- √ 1/8 cup coconut oil
- √ 1 sweet onion, chopped
- √ 1½ pounds ground beef
- √ 1 teaspoon Worcestershire sauce
- √ 2 teaspoons salt
- √ ¼ teaspoon pepper

Dairy-free

Preparation Time: 15 minutes

Cooking Time: 30 minutes

Servings: 6

Difficulty: Medium

- √ 1 teaspoon thyme
- √ ½ teaspoon rosemary
- √ ½ cup beef broth
- √ 2 cups mixed frozen vegetables

Topping:

- √ 3 large potatoes,boiled
- √ ½ cup vegan butter
- √ salt

Directions: Oven: 400°F -   9" × 13" baking dish

In a heated skillet, melt coconut oil and cook all ingredients for around 15 minutes. Thee onions will be added next and cook for 5–10 minutes until tender. Add all topping ingredients and mash it in another bowl.

The beef mixture must be placed in an even layer in the prepared baking dish. Spread mashed potatoes over the top of the beef mixture. Bake for 30 minutes.

Nutrition:

Calories: 291

Fat: 12.5g

Fiber: 8.8g

Carbs: 35.7g

Protein: 12.2g

42. Southern Peach Pie

Ingredients:

- √ 1 unbaked Basic Gluten-Free Pie

Filling:

- √ 8 large peaches
- √ 3⁄4 cup sugar
- √ 1 1⁄2 teaspoons lemon juice
- √ 1⁄4 cup plus 1 tablespoon sorghum flour

Dairy-free

Preparation Time: 40 minutes

Cooking Time: 40 minutes

Servings: 12

Difficulty: Medium

- √ 1 teaspoon vanilla extract
- √ 4 tablespoons butter, thinly sliced

Topping:

- √ Whipped cream or ice cream

Directions: Oven: 350° F

In a bowl or container, all filling ingredients must be combined and pour peach filling into one 9" gluten-free pie shell. Lay slices of butter evenly over the top of the filling. Bake the pie for 40 minutes. Serve with whipped cream or ice cream.

Nutrition:

Calories: 189

Fat: 12.5g

Fiber: 4.5g

Carbs: 19.7g

Protein: 2.7g

43. Pineapple Tarts

Ingredients:

Filling:

- √ 4 medium pineapples

Pastry:

- √ 2 cups almond flour
- √ 1 1/4 cups vegan butter
- √ 2 eggs, beaten
- √ 3 tablespoons cold water

For assembly:

- √ 1 egg
- √ 1 tablespoon water

Vegetarian-friendly

Preparation Time: 15 minutes

Cooking Time: 25-30 minutes

Servings: 6

Difficulty: Hard

Directions:

Blend pineapple until it becomes a little chunky. Cook pineapple until the pulp turns brown, and the moisture is mostly cooked out. If you prefer a slightly sweeter filling, add sugar to taste while the pineapple cooks down.

Cool the filling and roll into balls. Ball sizes will depend on how you plan to shape your tarts.

For the pastry:

By hand, cut the butter into the flour until it is mixed in. Add remaining ingredietns. The dough must then be chilled for about 30 minutes. Assembly and baking in oven (350°F).

Whisk the beaten egg and water together to make an egg wash.

Roll out dime-sized filling balls. Using a cookie cutter, cut circles and encase the filling. Close the edges and seams. Brush with egg wash for extra shininess. Let the tart bake for about 15 minutes.

Nutrition:

Calories: 198

Fat: 3.5g

Fiber: 8.5g

Carbs: 21.9g

Protein: 2.3g

44. Pear Tarte Tatin

Ingredients:

Filling:

- √ 2 tablespoons shortening
- √ 2 pounds pears
- √ 3⁄4 cup granulated sugar
- √ 2 tablespoons cornstarch

Other recipes:

- √ 1 recipe basic gluten-free pie crust, chilled but not rolled out

Dairy-free/ Vegetarian-friendly

Preparation Time: 35 minutes

Cooking Time: 50 minutes

Servings: 8

Difficulty: Medium

Directions: Oven: 400° F

In a heated skillet, cook filling ingrediens and cook for 15 minutes. Transfer the pear mixture to an ungreased 9-inch glass pie dish.

Roll out the chilled pie making the size bigger than the diameter of the pie pan. Remove the parchment paper and drape the crust over the pear mixture, then fold the crust edges around the pears and tuck them into the dish.Lert it bake for about 30 to 35 minutes.

Nutrition:

Calories: 198

Fat: 9.5g

Fiber: 3.1g

Carbs: 19.7g

Protein: 3.7g

45. Cherry Almond Clafoutis

Ingredients:

Dairy-free/ Vegetarian-friendly

√   15-ounce cherries

√   2 eggs

√   ⅓ cup almond milk

√   2 tablespoons canola oil

√   1 teaspoon almond extract

√   ⅓ cup almond flour

√   ½ cup sugar

√   ¼ teaspoon salt

Preparation Time: 10 minutes

Cooking Time: 35 minutes

Servings: 4

Difficulty: Medium

Topping:

√   1 tablespoon almonds

√   2 tablespoons powdered sugar

Directions: Oven: 375°F

Grease an 8-inch baking dish with 2-inch sides. Spread the cherries evenly on the bottom.

In a blender, process the remaining ingredients The batter must then be poured over the cherries then sprinkle with the almonds. Bake for 25 to 35 minutes and dust with the powdered sugar.

Nutrition:

Calories: 214

Fat: 11.5g

Fiber: 4.1g

Carbs: 31.2g

Protein: 3.4g

46. Almond and Pear Tart

Ingredients:

Crust:

- √ ½ cup almond flour
- √ ½ cup yellow cornmeal
- √ 5 tablespoons sliced almonds
- √ 2 tablespoons sugar
- √ ½ teaspoon xanthan gum
- √ ¼ teaspoon cinnamon
- √ ¼ teaspoon salt
- √ ¼ cup coconut oil
- √ ¼ cup almond milk

Filling:

- √ 2 medium pears
- √ 2 eggs
- √ ½ cup sugar
- √ ⅓ cup almond flour
- √ ¼ cup almond flour
- √ 1 tablespoon vegan butter
- √ 1 teaspoon almond extract
- √ ⅛ teaspoon salt
- √ Whipped topping or vanilla ice cream

Dairy-free/ Vegetarian-friendly

Preparation Time: 20 minutes

Cooking Time: 40 minutes

Servings: 10

Difficulty: Medium

Directions: Oven: 400°F

Make the crust: In a food processor, pulse all crust ingredients and firmly press the dough one inch up the sides of a 9-inch tart pan.

Make the filling: cut each pear half into ¼-inch wedges and arrange attractively in a concentric circle on the crust. In a medium bowl, combine remaining ingredients then pour evenly over the pears.

Let the tart bake for about 40 minutes. Serve with ice cream or whipped cream if you wish.

Nutrition:

Calories: 89

Fat: 8.8g

Fiber: 3.5g

Carbs: 31.7g

Protein: 1.9g

47. Double Crust Apple Pie

Ingredients:

Dairy-free/ Vegetarian-friendly

Crust:

√   1 recipe gluten-free pie crust, unbaked

Preparation Time: 40 minutes

Filling:

Cooking Time: 45 minutes

√   3 Granny Smith apples

Servings: 8

√   3 Fuji apples

Difficulty: Hard

√   ⅓ cup brown sugar

√   ¼ cup almond flour

√   1 tablespoon lemon juice

√   2 teaspoons cinnamon

√   ½ teaspoon nutmeg

Directions: Oven: 375°F

Prepare the pie crust and divide the dough into 2 portions, one slightly larger than the other. Cover the smaller portion with plastic wrap and set it aside. Roll the larger dough portion into a circle about 12 inches in diameter. Fit it into a 9-inch glass deep-dish pie plate. The dough will fall over the edges slightly.

The apples must sliced into ¼-inch-thick slices. Place them in a container or bowl then add in the other filling ingredients. Spoon the apple mixture into the crust.

Roll out the top crust to about 9 inches in diameter. Place it over the filling in the pie plate. Take the overlapping edge of the bottom crust and roll it over the edge of the top crust, crimping to secure. Use a good knife to slice several slits into the top crust. Let the apple pie bake for about 30 minutes.

Cool the pie completely before slicing.

Nutrition:

Calories: 201

Fat: 10.4g

Fiber: 4.1g

Carbs: 32.1g

Protein: 1.9g

48. PB &J Tart

Ingredients:

Dairy-free/ Vegan

CRUST

Preparation Time: 45 minutes

- √ 1½ cups almond flour
- √ 3 tablespoons arrowroot starch
- √ 3 tablespoons sugar
- √ ¼ teaspoon of salt
- √ ¼ cup maple syrup
- √ 3 tablespoons coconut oil
- √ 1 teaspoon vanilla extract

Cooking Time: 50 minutes

Servings: 10

Difficulty: Medium

FILLING

- √ ½ cup coconut milk
- √ 1 cup coconut cream
- √ ¾ cup peanut butter

- √ ½ cup vegan cream cheese
- √ ½ cup of sugar
- √ 2 tablespoons arrowroot starch
- √ 2 tablespoons maple syrup
- √ 1 teaspoon vanilla extract
- √ ½ teaspoon baking powder
- √ ¼ teaspoon of salt

BLACKBERRY-CHIA JAM

- √ 2 cups frozen blackberries
- √ Juice of ½ lemon
- √ ¼ cup maple syrup
- √ 2 tablespoons chia seeds

Directions: Oven: 350°F

In a container or bowl, mix all crust ingredients. Gather the dough into a ball and refrigerate for 30 minutes. Spray a 9-inch tart pan with cooking spray.

Roll the dough until about ¼ inch thick. Flip it onto the prepared tart pan, and carefully press it into the bottom; to make the filling, in a high-speed blender or food processor, combine all filling ingredients.

Pour the filling into the tart pan with the crust. Let the tart bake for about 45 to 50 minutes.

To make the blackberry-chia jam, in a medium saucepan over medium-high heat, combine and cook all ingrediens for 15 minutes.

Once the tart and jam have cooled, carefully spread the jam on top of the tart.

Nutrition:

Calories: 249

Fat: 9.4g

Fiber: 3.5g

Carbs: 34g

Protein: 8.4 g

49. Custard Mini Tarts

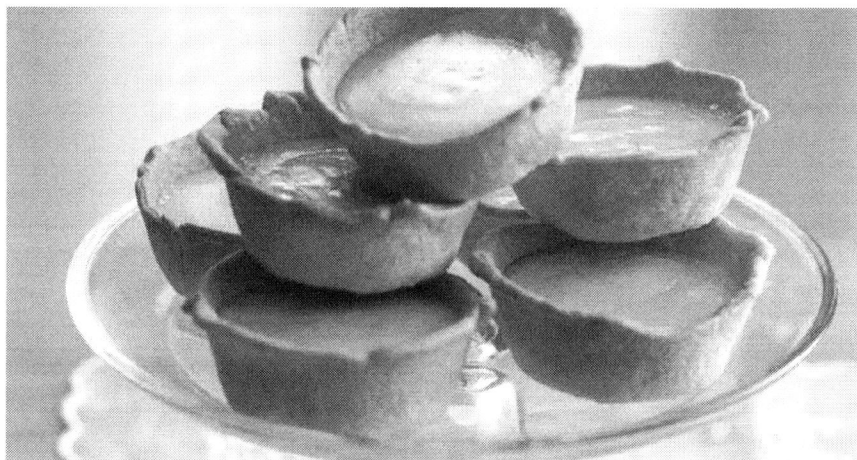

Ingredients:

CRUST

- √ 1½ cups almond flour
- √ 3 tablespoons arrowroot starch
- √ 3 tablespoons
- √ ¼ teaspoon of salt
- √ ¼ cup maple syrup
- √ 3 tablespoons coconut oil
- √ 1 teaspoon vanilla extract
- √ Nonstick cooking spray

CUSTARD

- √ 13.5-ounce coconut milk
- √ 2 teaspoons vanilla extract
- √ ½ cup maple syrup
- √ ¼ cup arrowroot starch

Dairy-free/ Vegan

Preparation Time: 20 minutes

Cooking Time: 25 minutes
Servings: 6
Difficulty: Medium

Directions: Oven: 350°F

In a container or bowl, mix all crust ingredients.Gather the dough into a ball and refrigerate for 30 minutes. Six 4-inch tart pans with removable bottoms will be sprayed with cooking spray. Roll the dough until about ¼ inch thick. Flip it onto the prepared tart pan, and carefully press it into the bottom.

To make the filling, in a high-speed blender or food processor, combine all filling ingredients. Pour the filling into the tart pan with the crust. Let the tart bake for about 25 minutes.

Nutrition:

Calories: 199

Fat: 5.5g

Fiber: 3.4g

Carbs: 29.7g

Protein: 1.8 g

50. Fig Apple Crumble

Ingredients:

CRUST

- √ 1¾ cups almond flour
- √ ¼ cup tapioca flour
- √ 3 tablespoons coconut sugar
- √ 2 teaspoons cinnamon
- √ ¼ teaspoon salt
- √ ¼ cup coconut oil
- √ ¼ cup maple syrup
- √ 1 teaspoon vanilla extract
- √ 1 teaspoon vinegar

FILLING

- √ 2 cups dried figs
- √ ¼ cup coconut oil
- √ 4 cups apples
- √ ¼ cup sugar
- √ Juice of ½ lemon
- √ 1 tablespoon cinnamon
- √ 1 teaspoon nutmeg
- √ 1 teaspoon vanilla extract

Dairy-free/ Vegan

Preparation Time: 45 minutes

Cooking Time: 50 minutes

Servings: 10

Difficulty: Hard

- √ ½ teaspoon allspice
- √ ⅛ teaspoon cloves
- √ ⅛ teaspoon of salt

CRUMBLE

- √ 1 cup almond flour
- √ ¼ cup of coconut sugar
- √ 1 tablespoon coconut flour
- √ 1 teaspoon cinnamon
- √ ⅓ cup vegan butter

Directions:

The crust: In a bowl or container, combine all dry ingredients. In another bowl or container, whisk all wet ingredients. In the flour mixture, add in the wet ingredients. And beat until a crumbly dough forms. Chill.

Oven: 350°F - A 9-Inch pie plate must then be lightly greased.

To start the filling, in a medium bowl, cover the figs with boiling water. Soak for 15 to 20 minutes, until soft. Drain, roughly chop and set aside.

Lay dough balls in between two sheets of parchment paper. Making use of a rolling pin, roll it out to ⅛ to ¼ inch thick. Flip the flattened dough across the prepared pie plate, using your fingers to press it into the bottom, fix any cracks, and seal around the edges.

Prebake the crust for 10 minutes, then set aside until ready to use.

To finish the filling, in a large pot, cook all the filling ingredients for 20 minutes.

Transfer the apple-fig mixture to the prebaked crust.

For making the crumble topping, in a container or bowl, combine the all ingredients, mixing until crumble forms. Sprinkle the crumble over the apple-fig mixture. Let it bake for about 20 to 24 minutes until the crumble has started to turn golden brown

Nutrition:

Calories: 171

Fat: 4.5g

Fiber: 5.1g

Carbs: 16,5g

Protein: 3.4g

51. Blueberry Pie

Ingredients:

CRUST

- √ 1¾ cups almond flour
- √ ¼ cup arrowroot starch
- √ 3 tablespoons coconut sugar
- √ 2 teaspoons ground cinnamon
- √ ¼ teaspoon of salt
- √ ¼ cup coconut oil
- √ ¼ cup maple syrup
- √ 1 teaspoon vanilla extract
- √ 1 teaspoon vinegar

FILLING

- √ ¼ cup coconut oil
- √ 4 cups blueberries
- √ ½ cup sugar
- √ Juice of ½ lemon
- √ 1 teaspoon vanilla extract
- √ 2 tablespoons arrowroot starch

CRUMBLE TOPPING

- √ 1 cup almond flour
- √ ¼ cup of coconut sugar
- √ ⅓ cup cold vegan butter

Dairy-free/ Vegan

Preparation Time: 20 minutes

Cooking Time: 25-30 minutes

Servings: 9

Difficulty: Medium

Directions: Oven: 350F - A 9-Inch pie plate must then be lightly greased.

Crust: In a bowl or container, mix all dry ingredients.

In another bowl or container, mix all wet ingredients.

In the flour mixture, add in the wet ingredients and beat until a crumbly dough forms. Chill.

Lay dough balls in between two sheets of parchment paper. Making use of a rolling pin, roll it out to ⅛ to ¼ inch thick. Flip the flattened dough across the prepared pie plate, using your fingers to press it into the bottom, fix any cracks, and seal around the edges.

Prebake the crust for 10 minutes, then set aside until ready to use.

To make the filling, in a large pot, cook all ingredients until the mixture has reduced and thickened. Transfer the blueberry mixture to the pie plate with the prebaked crust. Set aside.

To make the crumble topping, in another medium bowl, mix all ingredients until a crumbly dough form. Sprinkle the crumble over the blueberry mixture.

Let it bake for about 20 to 24 minutes, until the crust edges and crumble have started to turn golden brown.

Nutrition:

Calories: 201

Fat: 9.5g

Fiber: 4.1g

Carbs: 16.7g

Protein: 1.4g

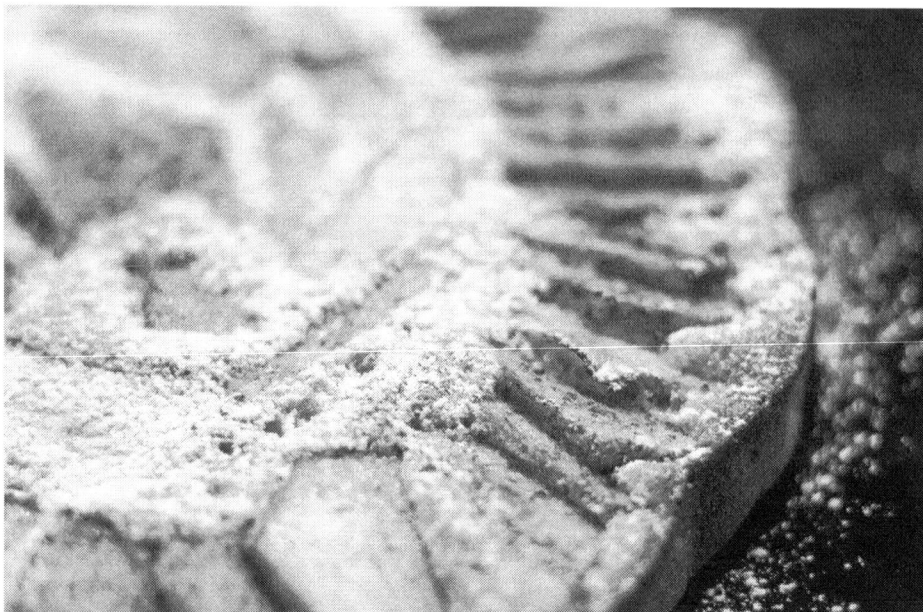

Chapter 5. <u>CUPCAKES AND MUFFINS</u>

52. Blueberry Muffins

Ingredients:

Wet:

- √ ¼ cup coconut oil
- √ 1 cup brown sugar
- √ 2 eggs
- √ 1 tsp. vanilla
- √ ½ cup sour cream
- √ ½ cup whole milk
- √ 1 tsp. lemon juice

Dry:

- √ ⅓ cup almond flour
- √ ½ cup brown rice flour
- √ ¼ cup sorghum flour
- √ 3 Tbsp. coconut flour
- √ ½ cup tapioca starch
- √ ½ cup potato starch
- √ 4 tsp. baking powder
- √ ½ tsp. gelatin powder
- √ 2 cups blueberries

Vegetarian-friendly

Preparation Time: 25 minutes

Cooking Time: 30 minutes

Servings: 6

Difficulty: Easy

Directions: Oven: 375°F

Whisk all wet ingredients together. Combine all dry ingredients and mix well. The two will be mixed. Fold in blueberries throughout batter. Making use of an ice cream scooper, dollop batter into greased jumbo muffin tins. Bake for 24–25 minutes.

Nutrition:

Calories: 195

Fat: 5.1g

Fiber: 3.1g

Carbs: 26.1g

Protein: 4.1 g

53. Chocolate and Peanut Butter Cupcakes

Ingredients:

Dry Ingredients:

- √ ⅓ cup almond flour
- √ ½ cup rice flour
- √ ¼ cup sorghum flour
- √ 3 T coconut flour
- √ ½ cup tapioca starch
- √ ½ cup potato starch
- √ 4 tsp. baking powder
- √ ½ tsp. gelatin powder
- √ 1¼ cup brown sugar

Wet Ingredients:

- √ 2 Tbsp. vegan butter/ avocado or coconut oil
- √ 2 eggs
- √ 1 tsp. vanilla
- √ 1½ cup sour cream
- √ 1 cup whole milk
- √ ⅔ cup peanut butter
- √ 1 cup raw dark chocolate chips

Vegetarian-friendly

Preparation Time: 15 minutes

Cooking Time: 20 minutes

Servings: 6

Difficulty: Easy

Directions: Oven: 375°F

Whisk all dry ingredients together. Combine all dry ingredients and mix well. The dry ingredients will be added gradually to the wet mixture. Mix until well blended. Fold in the chocolate chips throughout batter. Spoon batter into a greased cupcake tin. Let it bake for about 20 minutes.

Nutrition:

Calories: 191

Fat: 4.9g

Fiber: 3.5g

Carbs: 25.1g

Protein: 2.7g

54. Apple Streusel Muffins

Ingredients:

Dry Ingredients:

- √ 1 cup coconut flour
- √ 1 tsp. xantham gum
- √ ½ cup of sugar
- √ ¾ cup brown sugar
- √ 3 tsp. baking powder
- √ 3 tsp. cinnamon

Wet Ingredients:

- √ 1 cup milk
- √ 1 tsp. vanilla extract
- √ 1 cup coconut oil
- √ 4 large eggs
- √ 2 cups minced apples

Streusel Topping:

- √ ½ cup brown sugar
- √ ¼ cup of rice flour
- √ 2 tsp. cinnamon
- √ 1 tsp. water
- √ ¼ cup vegan butter

Vegetarian-friendly

Preparation Time: 25 minutes

Cooking Time: 25 minutes

Servings: 12

Difficulty: Easy

Directions: Oven: 375°F

In a container or bowl, put in the sifted dry ingredients. In a separate bowl or standing mixer, combine wet ingredients. The dry ingredients will be gradually added and mix until fully moist. Fill muffin cups to the top with batter.

In a bowl or container, combine all listed streusel topping ingredients. Sprinkle each muffin generously with streusel topping. Let the muffins bake for about 20–25 minutes.

Nutrition:

Calories: 225

Fat: 8.5g

Fiber: 2.4g

Carbs: 26.5g

Protein: 2.1 g

55. Cheesy Corn Bread Muffins

Ingredients:

Dairy-free/ Vegetarian-friendly

Wet Ingredients:

Preparation Time: 10 minutes

- √ 3 tablespoons coconut oil, melted
- √ 2 large eggs
- √ 1 cup almond milk
- √ ¼ cup honey

Cooking Time: 25 minutes
Servings: 12
Difficulty: Medium

Dry Ingredients:

- √ 1 teaspoon cornstarch
- √ ½ teaspoon salt
- √ ½ teaspoon baking soda
- √ 1 cup cornmeal
- √ ½ cup gluten-free flour

Other ingredients:

- √ ⅓ cup shredded Vegan cheese
- √ 1 jalapeño pepper, seeded and diced

Directions: Oven: 350°F

In a bowl or container, all dry ingredients must be combined. In another bowl or container, all wet ingredients must be mixed too. Combine both mixture. Stir in the Cheddar cheese.

Pour the mixture the prepared muffin cups. Top each muffin with a piece of jalapeño pepper. Let it bake for about 25 minutes.

Nutrition:

Calories: 245

Fat: 10.5g

Fiber: 9.5g

Carbs:31g

Protein: 4.3g

56. Sunflower Seed Butter Muffin

Ingredients:

Dry ingredients:

- √ 80 grams gluten free oats
- √ 155 grams gluten-free flour
- √ ½ cup of coconut sugar
- √ 1 tablespoon baking powder
- √ ½ teaspoon salt

Wet Ingredients:

- √ ½ cup sunflower seed butter
- √ ¼ teaspoon coconut oil
- √ 1¼ cups coconut milk
- √ 2 teaspoons vanilla extract
- √ ⅓ cup of chocolate chips

Dairy-free/ Vegan

Preparation Time: 10 minutes

Cooking Time: 20 minutes

Servings: 12

Difficulty: Easy

Directions: Oven: 375° F

In the food processor, put in the oats and pulse until they resemble a coarse flour. In a bowl or container, add all dry ingredients plus the ground oats. Stir all.

Put in all wet ingredients. The batter must be divided equally to the muffin cups. Sprinkle the tops with a few additional chocolate chips.

Let the muffins bake for about 20 minutes.

Nutrition:

Calories: 241

Fat: 11g

Fiber: 4.2g

Carbs: 33.1g

Protein: 5.6g

57. Cheddar and Chive Muffins

Ingredients:

- √ ¼ tablespoon coconut oil
- √ 225 grams gluten-free flour
- √ 4 teaspoons baking powder
- √ 1 tablespoon chives
- √ ¼ teaspoon salt
- √ ¼ teaspoon garlic powder
- √ ¾ cup milk
- √ 2 large eggs
- √ 2 tablespoons sunflower oil
- √ 2 teaspoons honey
- √ 2 teaspoons vinegar
- √ 1 cup shredded Cheddar cheese

Vegetarian-friendly

Preparation Time: 15 minutes

Cooking Time: 12 minutes

Servings: 5

Difficulty: Easy

Directions: Oven: 375°F

In a bowl or container, all listed ingredients must be combined. The batter must be divided equally to the muffin cups. Bake for 15 minutes.

Nutrition:

Calories: 224

Fat: 11.5g

Fiber: 4.3g

Carbs: 29.5g

Protein: 1.9g

58. Carrot Cupcakes

Ingredients:

Dry:

- √ 1 cup almond flour
- √ 1 cup coconut flour
- √ 2 tablespoons xanthan gum
- √ 1 tablespoon baking powder
- √ ½ tablespoon baking soda
- √ 1 teaspoon cinnamon
- √ 1 cup of sugar

Wet:

- √ ¾ cup cooking oil
- √ 3 tablespoons coconut oil
- √ 2 eggs
- √ ½ cup of water
- √ 1 tablespoon vanilla extract
- √ 3 cups grated carrots

Dairy-free

Preparation Time: 15 minutes

Cooking Time: 20 minutes

Servings: 12

Difficulty: Easy

Directions:

Oven: 350°F

In a bowl or container, combine all dry ingredients. Do the same with the wet ingredients in another bowl. Gradually incorporate the two mixture. Scoop the batter into the muffin cups and bake for 20 minutes.

Nutrition:

Calories: 241

Fat: 11.9g

Fiber: 3.8g

Carbs: 31.8g

Protein: 2.1 g

59. Chocolate Chip Muffins

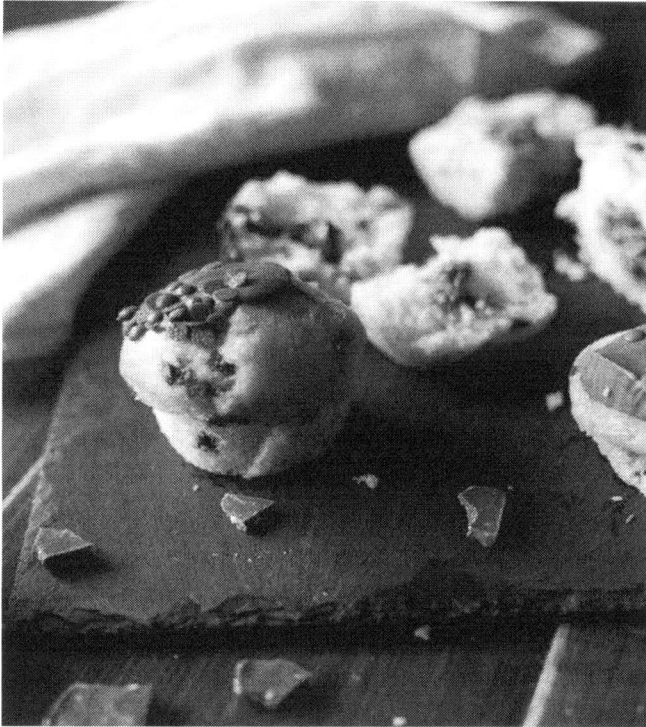

Ingredients:

- √ 1½ cups gluten-free flour
- √ 1 cup of sugar
- √ ½ teaspoon baking powder
- √ 1 teaspoon baking soda
- √ ¼ teaspoon salt
- √ 2 eggs
- √ 1 teaspoon vanilla extract
- √ ⅓ cup coconut oil
- √ 1 cup almond milk
- √ 1 cup dark chocolate chips

Dairy-free

Preparation Time: 15 minutes
Cooking Time: 25 minutes
Servings: 12
Difficulty: Easy

Directions: Oven: 350°F

In a bowl or container, all ingredients except the chocolate chips must be combined. Whisk until smooth. Fold in chocolate chips.

Scoop batter into prepared muffin tin. Let it bake for about 25 minutes.

Nutrition:

Calories: 243

Fat: 11.4g

Fiber: 4.4g

Carbs: 34g

Protein: 3.1g

60. Bacon and Egg Muffins

Ingredients:

√ Dry:

√ 2 cups gluten-free flour

√ ¼ cup of sugar

√ 1 tablespoon baking powder

√ ½ teaspoon baking soda

√ ½ teaspoon salt

Wet:

√ 2 eggs

√ 1 tablespoon vinegar

√ 1 cup almond milk

√ 1 cup of coconut oil

√ ½ cup chopped cooked bacon

Fillings:

√ 1 green onion, diced

√ 2 hard-boiled eggs, chopped

Topping:

√ 1/3 cup chopped cooked bacon

Dairy-Free

Preparation Time: 15 minutes

Cooking Time: 20 minutes

Servings: 12

Difficulty: Easy

Directions: Oven: 375F

In a bowl or container, combine both dry and wet ingredients. Fold in the fillings. Scoop batter into prepared muffin tin. Top with bacon bits. Bake for 20 minutes.

Nutrition:

Calories: 229

Fat: 12.2g

Fiber: 4.1g

Carbs: 22.4g

Protein: 1.9 g

61. Cinnamon Roll Muffins

Ingredients:

MUFFINS

- √ 1½ cups gluten-free flour
- √ ⅛ teaspoon salt
- √ ½ cup sugar
- √ 2 teaspoons baking powder
- √ ¾ cup almond milk
- √ egg
- √ 1 teaspoon vanilla extract
- √ ¼ cup coconut oil

TOPPING

- √ ¼ cupvegan butter
- √ ¼ cup brown sugar
- √ ½ tablespoon gluten-free flour
- √ ¾ teaspoon cinnamon

GLAZE

- √ cup confectioners' sugar
- √ 2½ tablespoons almond milk
- √ ½ teaspoon vanilla extract

Dairy-free

Preparation Time: 15 minutes

Cooking Time: 25 minutes

Servings: 12

Difficulty: Medium

Directions: Oven: 350°F

In a container, add all muffin ingredients and combine well. Scoop batter into prepared muffin tin.

In a separate bowl, cream the topping ingredients together. Drop a teaspoonful of topping on each muffin. Swirl the mixture by using a knife. Let it bake for about 25 minutes.

In a bowl or container, whisk the glaze ingredients together. Drizzle over warm muffins.

Nutrition:

Calories: 190

Fat: 6.5g

Fiber: 4.6g

Carbs: 31.7g

Protein: 1.9g

62. Vanilla Muffins

Ingredients:

Dry:

√ 1 cup Gluten-Free Flour

√ 1½ tsp baking powder

√ ⅛ tsp salt

√ ⅓ cup of sugar

Wet:

√ egg

√ ½ cup almond milk

√ tbsp coconut oil

√ 1 tsp vanilla

Dairy-free/ Vegetarian-friendly

Preparation Time: 15 minutes

Cooking Time: 18 minutes

Servings: 6

Difficulty: Easy

Directions: Oven: 400° F

In a container or bowl, combine all dry ingredients. Do the same with the wet ingredients. Combine both wet and dry ingredients. The batter must be poured into paper-lined muffin cups. Let it bake for around 15—18 minutes.

Nutrition:

Calories: 181

Fat: 4.5g

Fiber: 1.8g

Carbs: 29.9g

Protein: 1.2g

63. Lemon Poppy Seed Muffins

Ingredients:

Dry:

- √   ¼ cup of coconut flour
- √   1 tablespoon of poppy seeds
- √   1 tablespoon of lemon zest
- √   ¼ teaspoon of baking soda
- √   ¼ teaspoon of salt

Wet:

- √   3 eggs
- √   ¼ cup of agave
- √   ¼ teaspoon of lemon zest
- √   ¼ cup of grape seed oil

Dairy-free/ Vegetarian-friendly

Preparation Time: 15 minutes

Cooking Time: 8-10 minutes

Servings: 3

Difficulty: Easy

Directions:

In a container or bowl, combine all dry ingredients. Do the same with the wet ingredients. Combine both wet and dry ingredients.The batter must be poured into paper-lined muffin cups.and bake for 8-10 minutes.

Nutrition:

Calories: 169

Fat: 2.1g

Fiber: 3.1g

Carbs: 18.7g

Protein: 2.1g

64. Pumpkin Pie Cupcakes

Ingredients:

CUPCAKES

- √ 125 grams gluten-free flour
- √ 2 teaspoons pumpkin pie spice
- √ 1 teaspoon cinnamon
- √ ½ teaspoon xanthan gum
- √ ¼ teaspoon cloves
- √ ¼ teaspoon baking powder
- √ ¼ teaspoon baking soda
- √ ¼ teaspoon salt
- √ can coconut milk
- √ 150 grams granulated sugar
- √ eggs
- √ 1 (15-ounce) can pumpkin puree

COCONUT CREAM

- √ (14-ounce) can coconut cream, chilled overnight
- √ tablespoons powdered sugar

Dairy-free/ Vegetarian-friendly

Preparation Time: 15 minutes

Cooking Time: 30 minutes

Servings: 12

Difficulty: Easy

Directions:

Oven: 350F. A 12-cup muffin tin must be lined with cupcake liners.

In a bowl or container, whisk all cupcake ingredients to combine. The batter must be divided equally into prepared muffin cups. Let the cupcakes bake for 28 to 30 minutes.

COCONUT WHIPPED CREAM

A chilled can of coconut cream be opened. Pour off the watery liquid. Scoop only the solid part into a large bowl and add the powdered sugar. Using a handheld electric mixer, beat until smooth and creamy. Transfer to a piping bag with a star tip and apply some to each cupcake.

Nutrition:

Calories: 241

Fat: 11.5g

Fiber: 4.2g

Carbs: 33.1g

Protein: 2g

65. Gingerbread Cupcakes

Ingredients:

Vegetarian-friendly

- √ 167 grams gluten-free flour
- √ 2 tablespoons arrowroot
- √ 1½ teaspoons cinnamon
- √ ½ teaspoon xanthan gum
- √ ½ teaspoon baking powder
- √ ½ teaspoon baking soda
- √ ½ teaspoon ground ginger
- √ ½ teaspoon nutmeg
- √ ½ teaspoon cloves
- √ ¼ teaspoon salt
- √ ½ cup canola oil
- √ 100 grams t brown sugar
- √ ½ cup coconut milk
- √ ½ cup maple syrup
- √ egg
- √ 1 teaspoon vanilla extract
- √ ½ teaspoon vinegar

Preparation Time: 25 minutes

Cooking Time: 22 minutes

Servings: 12

Difficulty: Medium

CREAM CHEESE FROSTING

- √ 102 grams shortening
- √ 4 ounces non-dairy cream cheese
- √ 480 grams of powdered sugar
- √ teaspoon vanilla extract
- √ 4 tablespoons coconut milk

Directions: Oven: 350°F - Line a 12-cup muffin tin with cupcake liners.

In a bowl or container, combine all cupcake ingredients The batter must be divided equally to the muffin cups filling them two-thirds full. Let the cupcakes Bake for about 20 to 22 minutes.

CREAM CHEESE FROSTING

In a bowl or container, cream the cream cheese and shortening together. Add the powdered sugar and vanilla. Mix as you add the milk by the tablespoon until smooth and creamy.

Frost the cupcakes.

Nutrition:

Calories: 243

Fat: 9.9g

Fiber: 3.5g

Carbs: 31.9g

Protein: 2.5 g

66. Strawberry Cupcakes

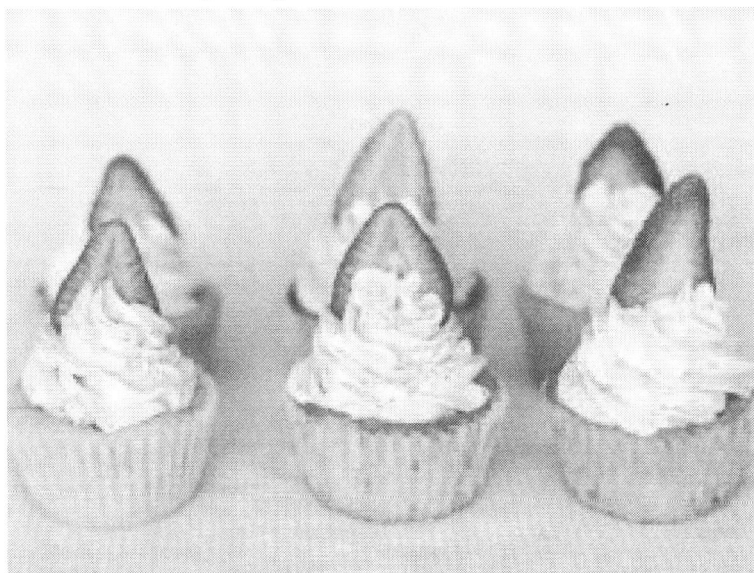

Ingredients:

FOR THE STRAWBERRY FILLING

- √ 250 grams strawberries
- √ 2 tablespoons granulated sugar

FOR THE CUPCAKES

Preparation Time: 45 minutes

Cooking Time: 40 minutes

Servings: 12

Difficulty: Hard

- √ 207 grams gluten-free flour
- √ 2 tablespoons arrowroot
- √ 1 teaspoon xanthan gum
- √ 1 teaspoon baking soda
- √ ¼ teaspoon salt
- √ 8 tablespoons coconut oil
- √ 200 grams white sugar
- √ 3 egg whites
- √ 60 grams Greek yogurt
- √ teaspoons vanilla extract
- √ ⅓ cup coconut milk

STRAWBERRY FROSTING

- √ 34 grams freeze-dried strawberries
- √ 240 grams of powdered sugar
- √ 68 grams shortening
- √ 2 to 3 tablespoons coconut milk
- √ teaspoon vanilla extract

Directions:

TO MAKE THE STRAWBERRY FILLING

In a small saucepan, combine the strawberries and sugar. Simmer over heat that is medium and cook for about 20 minutes, occasionally stirring to prevent burning.

CUPCAKES

Oven: 350F A 12-cup muffin tin will be lined with cupcake liners.

In a bowl or container, mix all cupcake ingredients. The batter must be divided equally to the muffin cups filling each two-thirds full. Let the cupcakes Bake for about 20 to 22 minutes.

TO MAKE THE STRAWBERRY FROSTING

In a food processor, pulse the freeze-dried strawberries to form a fine powder.

In a bowl or container, beat together the powdered sugar, shortening, strawberry powder, milk, and vanilla until smooth. The filling will then be transferred to a piping bag. Frost the cupcakes. Serve.

Nutrition:

Calories: 225

Fat: 11.4g

Fiber: 4.2g

Carbs: 33.1g

Protein: 3.1 g

Chapter 6. <u>COOKIES</u>

67. Snickerdoodles

Ingredients:

Dry:

- √ ⅓ cup almond flour
- √ 1 cup rice flour
- √ ½ cup sorghum flour
- √ ½ cup tapioca starch
- √ ¼ cup potato starch
- √ Tbsp. Corn starch
- √ ½ tsp. gelatin powder
- √ tsp. Baking powder
- √ ½ tsp. Salt
- √ ½ tsp. cinnamon
- √ 1 cup brown sugar
- √ ½ cup of sugar

Wet:

- √ egg
- √ Tbsp. sour cream
- √ 1 tsp. vanilla extract
- √ 1½ cup coconut oil

FOR ROLLING

- √ ⅓ cup sugar
- √ tsp. cinnamon

Vegetarian-friendly

Preparation Time: 45 minutes

Cooking Time: 10 minutes

Servings: 6

Difficulty: Medium

Directions: Oven: 350°F

In a container or bowl, combine all dry ingredients. Do the same with the wet ingredients. Combine both wet and dry ingredients gradually. Form into a dough.

The dough must be frozen for 30 minutes. Mix remaining sugar and cinnamon together. Make balls out of the dough and then into the cinnamon-sugar mixture to coat. Place dough balls on the cookie sheet and let the cookies bake for 8–10 minutes.

Nutrition:

Calories: 101

Fat: 3.5g

Fiber: 1.3g

Carbs: 10.7g

Protein: 1.2g

68. Cranberry Cookies

Ingredients:

Vegetarian-friendly

- √ 1 cup avocado oil
- √ 1½ cups powdered sugar
- √ 1 tsp. vanilla extract
- √ 1 egg
- √ ⅔ cups almond flour
- √ cup rice flour
- √ ⅔ cups sorghum flour
- √ ⅔ cups tapioca starch
- √ ⅓ cup potato starch
- √ tsp. baking powder
- √ 1½ tsp. gelatin powder
- √ ½ tsp. Salt

Preparation Time: 15 minutes

Cooking Time: 12 minutes

Servings: 6

Difficulty: Easy

Other ingredients:

- √ 1½ cups coconut flakes
- √ 1½ cups dried cranberries

Directions: Oven: 350°F

Using a stand mixture, cream together butter, sugar, vanilla, and egg. Combine all remaining ingredients except coconut flakes and cranberries and mix well.

The dry and wet ingredients will then be combined. Add coconut and mix well. Fold in dried cranberries. Using a cookie scoop, place dough on a baking sheet and flatten slightly with the back of a spoon. Bake for 12 minutes.

Nutrition:

Calories: 111

Fat: 2.8g

Fiber: 5.8g

Carbs: 12.2g

Protein: 1.3g

69. Lemon Cookies

Ingredients:

Dairy-free/ Vegan

- √ 6 tablespoons water
- √ 2 tablespoons flaxseed meal

Preparation Time: 15 minutes

Cooking Time: 14 minutes

Dry:

Servings: 12

- √ 2¼ cups Gluten-Free Flour
- √ teaspoon baking powder
- √ 1 teaspoon baking soda
- √ 1 teaspoon gelatin powder
- √ 1/4 teaspoon salt

Difficulty: Easy

Wet:

- √ cup oil
- √ 3/4 cup white sugar
- √ 3/4 cup brown sugar
- √ 1 tablespoon lemon extract
- √ Lemon Zest

Directions: Oven: 350°F

In a bowl or container, combine the water and flaxseed meal and allow to thicken for 3 to 5 minutes. In another container, combine all dry ingredients.

Then in a third container, cream the oil and sugars together then pour in remaining ingredients and the flaxseed meal mixture, and beat the batter again until it is fluffy Combine it with the dry mixture.

Utilizing an ice cream scooper, drop the dough onto the prepared baking sheets. Bake for 14 minutes.

Nutrition:

Calories: 184

Fat: 11.5g

Fiber: 5.1g

Carbs: 22.9g

Protein: 1.9 g

70. Chewy Maple Cookies

Ingredients:

√ 3 tablespoons water

√ 1 tablespoon ground flaxseed meal

√ 1¾ cups Gluten-Free All-Purpose Flour

√ 2 teaspoons baking powder

√ 1⁄2 teaspoon gelatin powder

√ 1⁄4 teaspoon salt

√ cup brown sugar

√ 1⁄2 cup oil

√ 1⁄2 cup maple syrup

√ 1⁄2 teaspoon vanilla extract

√ 1⁄2 cup sweetened flaked coconut

Dairy-free/ Vegan

Preparation Time: 20 minutes

Cooking Time: 12 minutes

Servings: 12

Difficulty: Easy

Directions: Oven: 350° F.

In a bowl or container, combine the flaxseed meal and water, allow to thicken for 3 to 5 minutes. In another container, combine all dry ingredients.

Then in a third container, cream the oil and sugars together then pour in remaining ingredients and the flaxseed meal mixture, and beat the batter again until it is fluffy Combine it with the dry mixture. Fold in the coconut. Utilizing an ice cream scooper, drop the dough 2 inches apart onto the prepared baking sheets. Let it bake for about 12 minutes.

Nutrition:

Calories: 184

Fat: 8.9g

Fiber: 3.5g

Carbs: 24.7g

Protein: 2.9 g

71. Raisin Oatmeal Cookies

Ingredients:

Wet:

- √ ¾ cup brown sugar
- √ ¼ cup of sugar
- √ ¾ cup coconut oil
- √ ¼ cup milk
- √ 2 large eggs
- √ tsp. vanilla extract

Dry:

- √ cup rice flour
- √ 1 tsp. cinnamon
- √ ½ tsp. baking soda
- √ ¼ tsp. salt
- √ cups gluten-free oats
- √ 1 cup raisins

Vegetarian-friendly

Preparation Time: 30 minutes

Cooking Time: 15 minutes

Servings: 12

Difficulty: Easy

Directions: Oven: 350°F

In a bowl or container, cream sugars and oil until smooth. Add in other wet ingredients.

In a separate bowl, combine dry ingredients. Combine both mixture. Drop by the spoonful ontocookie sheets. Bake for 15 minutes.

Nutrition:

Calories: 199

Fat: 10.1g

Fiber: 3.5g

Carbs: 26.5g

Protein: 2.1g

72. Avocado Cream Cheese Cookies

Ingredients:

Wet:

- √ ⅓ cup coconut oil
- √ ½ avocado
- √ ½ pkg. cream cheese
- √ ½ cup sugar
- √ 2 Tbsp. lemon juice

Dry:

- √ tsp. Poppy seeds
- √ ½ almond flour
- √ ½ cup rice flour
- √ ½ tsp. baking soda

Vegetarian-friendly

Preparation Time: 25 minutes

Cooking Time: 15 minutes
Servings: 12
Difficulty: Easy

Directions: Oven: 375°F

Cream all wet ingredients together then add in all dry ingredients. Stir well. Insert a star tip in the piping bag and fill with cookie batter and pipe out cookies onto the prepared trays.Let the cookies bake for 15 minutes.

Nutrition:

Calories: 189

Fat: 11.1g

Fiber: 4.1g

Carbs: 11.7g

Protein: 1.4g

73. Best Chocolate Chip Cookies

Ingredients:

Wet:

- √ egg or 1 tablespoon ground flaxseeds mixed with 2 tablespoons warm water
- √ 1/4 cup Shortening

Dairy-free/ Vegan

Preparation Time: 20 minutes

Cooking Time: 10 minutes

- √ 1/4 cup white sugar
- √ 3/4 cup brown sugar
- √ tablespoon vanilla extract

Dry:

- √ 1/2 cup tapioca starch
- √ 3/4 cup sorghum flour
- √ 1/2 teaspoon sea salt
- √ 1/4 teaspoon agar-agar
- √ teaspoon baking powder
- √ 1/2 teaspoon baking soda

Other ingredients:

- √ cup semisweet chocolate chips

Servings: 12
Difficulty: Easy

Directions: Oven: 375°F

In a bowl or container, cream together all wet ingredients. In another container or bow, dry ingredients must be whisked together. Carefully combine the two mixture. Stir chocolate chips. Drop batter onto lined baking sheets. Let the cookies bake for 10 minutes.

Nutrition:

Calories: 191

Fat: 9.5g

Fiber: 5.4g

Carbs: 22.7g

Protein: 1.3g

74. Spiced Cookies

Ingredients:

Dry:

- √ 1½ cups gluten-free flour
- √ 1 teaspoon xanthan gum
- √ ½ teaspoon baking soda
- √ ¼ teaspoon salt½ teaspoon cinnamon

Vegetarian-friendly

Preparation Time: 25 minutes

Cooking Time: 25 minutes

Servings: 24

Difficulty: Medium

- √ ¼ teaspoon nutmeg
- √ ⅛ teaspoon cloves

Wet:

- √ ¼ cup coconut oil
- √ ¼ cup brown sugar
- √ ⅓ cup granulated sugar
- √ 2 teaspoons vanilla extract
- √ egg

Directions: Oven: 350°F.

In a bowl or container, put in all dry ingredients.

In a bowl or container, beat the oil with sugars. Add in remaining wet ingedients. The dough must be wrapped tightly in plastic wrap and chill for 1 hour. Drop by tablespoonfuls on the baking sheet. Bake until firm, 10 to 12 minutes.

Nutrition:

Calories: 190

Fat: 10.5g

Fiber: 4.2g

Carbs: 19.5g

Protein: 1.4g

75. Chocolate Chip Oatmeal Cookies

Ingredients:

Wet:

- √ 8 tablespoons coconut oil
- √ ½ cup granulated sugar
- √ ½ cup brown sugar
- √ 2 large eggs
- √ ½ teaspoon vanilla extract

Dairy-free/ Vegetarian-friendly

Preparation Time: 15 minutes

Cooking Time: 10 minutes

Servings: 18

Difficulty: Easy

Dry:

- √ teaspoon cinnamon
- √ ½ teaspoon salt
- √ ½ teaspoon baking soda
- √ ⅔ cup almond flour

Other Ingredients:

- √ 3 cups gluten-free oats
- √ ½ cup of chocolate chips

Directions: Oven: 350°F

In a bowl or container, beat together the sugar and butter. Add in the eggs one at a time and cream together. Stir in the remaining wet and dry ingredients. Fold in the oats and chocolate chips. Spoonful's of the dough must be dropped onto sheet pans. Let it bake for about 12 minutes.

Nutrition:

Calories: 190

Fat: 11.2g

Fiber: 4.1g

Carbs: 20g

Protein: 1.2g

76. Double Chocolate Chip Cookies

Ingredients:

Dairy-free/ Vegetarian-friendly

- √ 2½ cups confectioners' sugar
- √ ½ cup cocoa powder
- √ ¼ teaspoon cinnamon
- √ ½ teaspoon salt
- √ 3 large egg whites
- √ teaspoon vanilla extract
- √ 2½ cups chocolate chips

Preparation Time: 15 minutes

Cooking Time: 10 minutes

Servings: 18

Difficulty: Easy

Directions: Oven: 350°F.

In a bowl or container, combine all dry ingredients. Stir in the vanilla extract and egg whites. Fold in the chocolate chips. Drop tablespoons of batter ontosheet pans. Let the cookies Bake for about 15 to 17 minutes.

Nutrition:

Calories: 178

Fat: 10.5g

Fiber: 4g

Carbs: 18.4g

Protein: 1.2g

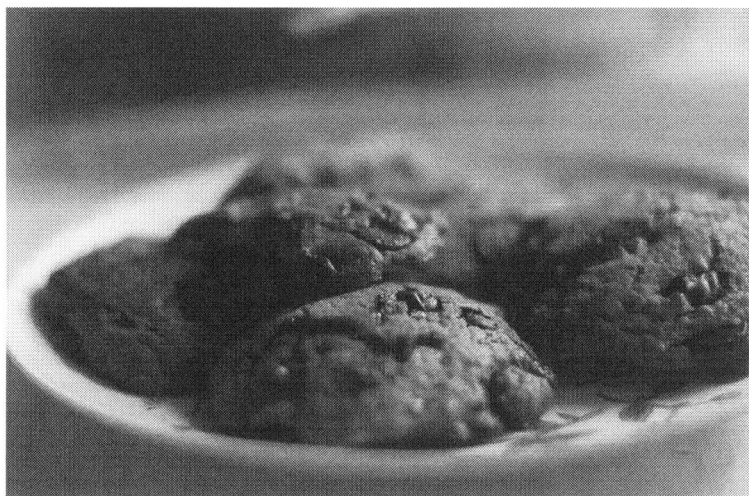

77. Ginger Cookies

Ingredients:

- √ 240 grams gluten-free flour
- √ ¾ cup granulated sugar
- √ 2 teaspoons ginger powder
- √ 1 teaspoon cinnamon
- √ ½ teaspoon nutmeg
- √ ¼ teaspoon salt
- √ egg
- √ ¼ cup palm shortening
- √ teaspoon vanilla extract

Dairy-free/ Vegetarian-friendly

Preparation Time: 15 minutes

Cooking Time: 10 minutes

Servings: 12

Difficulty: Easy

Directions: Oven: 350°F

In a bowl or container, whisk all the ingredients. Stir until the batter is smooth. Scoop tablespoonful of batter onto the baking sheet. Bake for 8 to 10 minutes.

Nutrition:

Calories: 190

Fat: 12g

Fiber: 4.1g

Carbs: 19.5g

Protein: 1.2g

78. Red Velvet Whoopie Pies

Ingredients:

Vegetarian-friendly

PIES

Preparation Time: 30 minutes

- √ 250 grams gluten-free flour
- √ 15 grams cocoa powder
- √ 1 teaspoon baking soda
- √ ½ teaspoon xanthan gum
- √ ½ teaspoon salt
- √ 8 tablespoons coconut oil
- √ 200 grams brown sugar
- √ egg
- √ ⅔ cup coconut milk
- √ teaspoons vanilla extract
- √ ½ teaspoon vinegar
- √ 1 teaspoon red food coloring

Cooking Time: 8 minutes
Servings: 12
Difficulty: Hard

FILLING

- √ 51 grams shortening
- √ 4 ounces cream cheese
- √ tablespoon coconut milk
- √ 1 teaspoon vanilla extract
- √ 300 grams of powdered sugar

Directions: Oven: 375°F

Pies: In a bowl or container, all dry ingredients must be combined.

In another bowl or container, cream together the oil and sugar. Add the egg and vanilla.Beat in the two mixture to form a dough. Roll the dough into balls and place them on the baking pan. Bake for 8 minutes. Meanwhile, combine all filling ingredients. Put in between two cooled pies.

Nutrition:

Calories: 191

Fat: 11.1g

Fiber: 4.9g

Carbs: 20.1g

Protein: 1.0g

79. Peanut Butter Cookies

Ingredients:

Wet:

- √ ½ cup white sugar
- √ ½ cup brown sugar
- √ ½ cup shortening
- √ tbsp water
- √ ½ cup peanut butter
- √ 1 egg

Dry:

- √ 1½ cup Gluten-Free Flour
- √ ½ tsp baking powder
- √ ¾ tsp baking soda
- √ ¼ tsp salt

Dairy-free

Preparation Time: 15 minutes

Cooking Time: 10 minutes

Servings: 24

Difficulty: Medium

Directions: Oven: 375°F.

Combine all wet ingredients until well combined.

The dry ingredients must be added until it forms a dough.

Measure dough by tablespoons, roll into 1" balls and place on an ungreased cookie sheet. Lightly flatten dough balls with a fork that has been dipped in sugar or flour, in a crisscross pattern. Let it bake for about 8—10 minutes.

Nutrition:

Calories: 191

Fat: 10.1g

Fiber: 4.1g

Carbs: 29.2g

Protein: 3.1g

80. Caramel Apple Cookies

Ingredients:

COOKIES:

- √ ½ cup coconut oil
- √ 6.75 oz gluten-free flour
- √ 2 tablespoons almond milk
- √ ¾ teaspoon baking soda
- √ ¼ teaspoon salt
- √ 2 tablespoons almond milk
- √ ½ cup rice flour
- √ 1 large egg
- √ ½ cup brown sugar
- √ ¾ teaspoon vanilla extract
- √ 1 pc apple slices

CARAMEL:

- √ 20 caramel candies
- √ 2 tablespoons water

Dairy-free/ Vegetarian- friendly

Preparation Time: 30 minutes

Cooking Time: 20 minutes

Servings: 12

Difficulty: Medium

Directions: Oven: 325°F.

Cream oil and sugar together then add in all remaining ingredients for the cookies. Fold in apple slices.

Roll dough into balls, tablespoon each, then bake for 14 minutes Place water and caramel candies in a small size saucepan and cook over low heat while stirring to smoothen for 7 minutes. Remove from heat and drizzle glaze over the cookies.

Nutrition:

Calories: 191

Fat: 8.1g

Fiber: 4.1g

Carbs: 30.1g

Protein: 3.1g

81. Thumbprint Cookies

Ingredients:

- √ 3 tablespoons water
- √ 1 tablespoon ground flaxseed meal
- √ 2 1/4 cups gluten free flour
- √ 1 1/2 teaspoons ground cinnamon
- √ teaspoon baking soda
- √ 1 teaspoon baking powder
- √ 1 teaspoon salt
- √ teaspoon agar-agar powder
- √ 1/2 teaspoon nutmeg
- √ 1/4 teaspoon allspice
- √ 1/4 teaspoon cloves
- √ 1 cup oil
- √ 3/4 cup brown sugar
- √ 3/4 cup granulated sugar
- √ teaspoon vanilla extract
- √ 1/2– 3/4 cup apricot or strawberry jam

Dairy-free/ Vegan

Preparation Time: 40 minutes

Cooking Time: 10-12 minutes

Servings: 24

Difficulty: Medium

Directions: Oven: 325°F. Line 2 baking sheets with parchment paper.

In a bowl or container, combine the flaxseed meal and water, allow to thicken for 3 to 5 minutes. In another bowl or container, add all dry ingredients

In a third bowl or container, combine all wet ingredients. Combine in the flaxseed mixture and dry micture. Roll each tablespoon of dough into a ball. Place the balls on the baking sheets. Using the tip of your thumb or finger, press a light indentation into the top of each ball and put 1/2 teaspoon of the jam of your choice. Bake for 12 minutes.

Nutrition:

Calories: 169

Fat: 5.5g

Fiber: 8.5g

Carbs: 27.5g

Protein: 2.6 g

82. Sugar Cookies

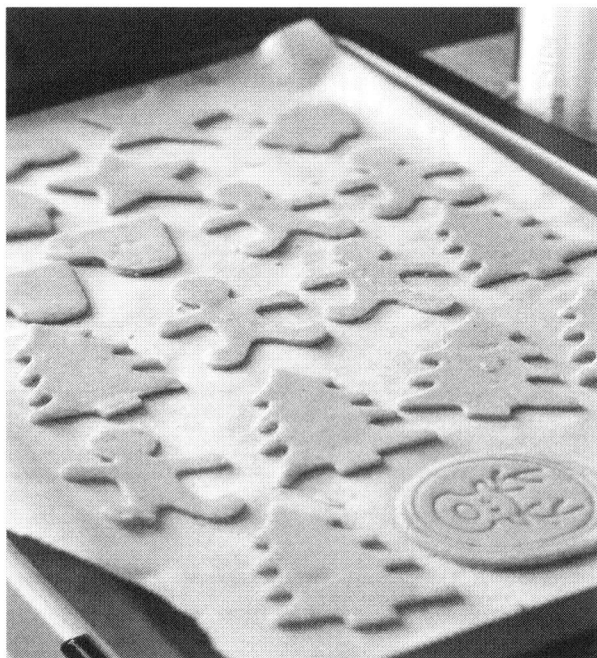

Ingredients:

- √ ⅓ cup coconut oil
- √ 1 egg yolk
- √ ½ cup of sugar
- √ 2 teaspoons vanilla extract
- √ 2 teaspoons lemon zest

Vegetarian-friendly/ Dairy-free

Preparation Time: 16 minutes

Cooking Time: 10 minutes

Servings: 24

Difficulty: Easy

- √ 1½ cups Gluten-Free Flour
- √ ¼ cup cornstarch
- √ ¼ teaspoon xanthan gum
- √ ¼ teaspoon salt
- √ ⅛ teaspoon baking soda
- √ 2 tablespoons water
- √ Rice flour, for rolling

Directions: Oven: 375°F

Using a food processor, combine all ingredients.Shape into two flat disks and wrap tightly. Refrigerate for 2 hours. Working with one disk of dough, roll with a rolling pin to ¼ inch thick on a sheet of parchment paper sprinkled with rice flour. Cut into shapes you like and transfer to a baking sheet Bake for 10 minutes.

Nutrition:

Calories: 199

Fat: 12g

Fiber: 4.4g

Carbs: 21g

Protein: 1.4g

83. Almond Biscotti

Ingredients:

- √ 1 cup gluten-free flour
- √ ¾ cup almond meal
- √ ½ cup potato starch
- √ 2 teaspoons baking powder
- √ 2 teaspoons xanthan gum
- √ teaspoon salt
- √ 3 eggs
- √ ⅔ cup brown sugar
- √ teaspoon almond extract

Dairy-free/ Vegetarian-friendly

Preparation Time: 25 minutes

Cooking Time: 1 hr. and 5 minutes

Servings: 22

Difficulty: Hard

Coating:

- √ 2 cups chocolate chips
- √ cup chopped almonds

Directions: Oven: 325°F

The baking sheet must be lined with parchment then set it aside. In a bowl or container, mix all dry ingredients.

In another bowl or container, whisk other remaining ingredients This will be added to the flour mixture and stir to form a dough.

Turn the dough onto the prepared baking sheet and cut in half. Form each half into an 11-by-4-inch log. Bake until slightly browned, 30 to 35 minutes.

Cut the logs into 1-inch-thick diagonal slices. Bake until slightly browned, another 25 to 30 minutes.

In a shallow glass bowl, microwave the chocolate chunks on high for 30 to 60 seconds, just until starting to melt. Stir to melt completely. Dip each side of the biscotti into the melted chocolate. Sprinkle with the chopped almonds.

Nutrition:

Calories: 180

Fat: 9.5g

Fiber: 4.1g

Carbs: 21.7g

Protein: 1.2g

84. Thin Mint Cookies

Ingredients:

COOKIES

- √ 190 grams gluten-free flour
- √ 75 grams cocoa powder
- √ 1 teaspoon baking powder
- √ ½ teaspoon xanthan gum
- √ ¼ teaspoon salt

Dairy-free/ Vegetarian-friendly

Preparation Time: 15 minutes

Cooking Time: 10 minutes

Servings: 28

Difficulty: Medium

- √ 179 grams shortening
- √ 200 grams sugar
- √ large egg
- √ teaspoon vanilla extract
- √ ¼ teaspoon peppermint extract

COATING

- √ 360 grams chocolate chips
- √ ½ teaspoon coconut oil
- √ ¼ teaspoon peppermint extract

Directions: Oven: 350°F

Line 2 baking sheets with parchment paper. In a bowl or container, all dry ingredients must be combined.

In a container or bowl, cream together all wet ingredients. Next, combine the flour mixture. Roll the dough to a large roundabout ¼ inch thick. Using a 2-inch round cookie cutter, cut out the cookies and place them on the baking sheets. Bake for 8 to 10 minutes.

TO MAKE THE COATING

In a medium saucepan, melt all listed ingredients. Dip each cookie in the melted chocolate and coat completely. Making use of a fork, lift each out of the chocolate, letting any excess fall back into the pan. Place the dipped cookies back on the parchment-lined baking sheets. Refrigerate for 30 minutes.

Nutrition:

Calories: 197

Fat: 13g

Fiber: 4.9g

Carbs: 22.7g

Protein: 1.9g

85. Linzer Cookies

Ingredients:

- √ 1 1/4 cups brown rice flour
- √ 3/4 cup arrowroot starch
- √ 3 tablespoons almond flour

Dairy-free/ Vegetarian-friendly

Preparation Time: 40 minutes

Cooking Time: 15 minutes

Servings: 12

- √ 1 teaspoon salt
- √ teaspoon xanthan gum
- √ 1 teaspoon lemon zest
- √ 6 tablespoons Shortening
- √ 1 1/4 cups sugar
- √ 2 large eggs
- √ teaspoon vanilla extract
- √ Confectioners' sugar
- √ 10-ounce strawberry jam

Difficulty: Hard

Directions: Oven: 350°F. The baking sheet must be lined with parchment then set it aside.

In a bowl or container, all dry ingredients must be combined. In other bowl or container, cream together all wet ingredients. Add dry ingredients 1/2 cup at a time and stir together into a stiff dough. Roll out cookies between 1/4" and 1/2" thickness and cut out using circle cookie cutters. Make sure to cut out two cookies for each Linzer "sandwich." You'll have one regular cut-out cookie and another cookie in the same shape, but with a hole in the center made from the smaller nesting cookie cutter. When the cookies are assembled, you'll see the jam between the layers.

Place cookies on lined cookie sheets and bake for 12–15 minutes Dust cookies with powdered sugar. Spread 1–2 teaspoons jam over the bottom cookie layer and then add the top cookie.

Nutrition:

Calories: 150

Fat: 1.5g

Fiber: 4.5g

Carbs: 12.7g

Protein: 1.7g

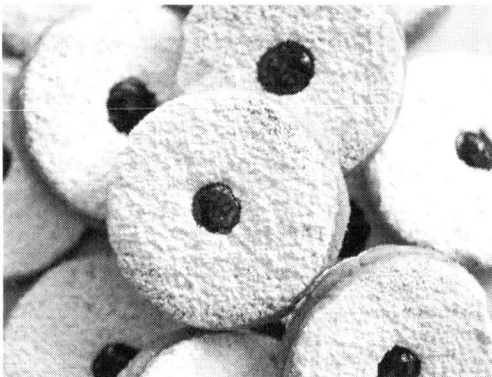

Chapter 7. <u>BROWNIES AND BARS</u>

86. Chocolate Mint Brownies

Ingredients:

BROWNIE

- √ ¼ cup almond flour
- √ ¼ cup sorghum flour
- √ ¼ cup coconut flour
- √ ¼ cup tapioca starch
- √ ¼ cup potato starch
- √ ½ cup cacao powder
- √ ½ tsp. gelatin powder
- √ ⅛ tsp. Salt
- √ 2 cups of sugar
- √ ½ cup of coconut oil
- √ 5 eggs

MINT FILLING

- √ 2 cups powdered
- √ sugar
- √ ½ cup vegan butter softened
- √ Tbsp. Milk
- √ ½ tsp. gluten-free mint extract

CHOCOLATE TOPPING

- √ 2 cups chocolate chips
- √ 8 Tbsp. vegan butter
- √ tsp. mint extract

Vegetarian-friendly

Preparation Time: 15 minutes

Cooking Time: 30 minutes

Servings: 6

Difficulty: Medium

Directions: Oven: 350°F.

Using a stand mixer, cream together sugar and coconut oil. Mix in eggs one at a time. Combine all the remaining dry ingredients. Pour batter into a greased a 9 × 13 baking pan. Bake for 30 minutes.

Combine all the ingredients for the filling and mix until smooth and creamy. Spread over the top of the cooled brownies. Refrigerate for a few minutes to set while making chocolate topping.

In a saucepan, melt butter and chocolate chips. When completely melted, add mint extract and blend in well. Spread chocolate topping over the filling.

Nutrition:

Calories: 258

Fat: 11.5g

Fiber: 12.1g

Carbs: 29.1g

Protein: 6.1g

87. Strawberry Bars

Ingredients:

Vegetarian-friendly

- √ ½ cup brown rice flour
- √ ½ cup white rice flour
- √ ⅓ cup sorghum flour
- √ ¼ cup almond flour
- √ ½ cup tapioca starch
- √ ½ cup potato starch
- √ tsp. gelatin powder
- √ ½ tsp. baking powder
- √ ½ cup of sugar
- √ ½ cup brown sugar
- √ cup coconut oil
- √ 1 egg
- √ 1 cup chopped nuts
- √ 10-oz. strawberry jam
- √ ¼ cup gluten-free oats

Preparation Time: 30 minutes

Cooking Time: 40 minutes

Servings: 8

Difficulty: Easy

Directions: Oven: 350°F.

Using a stand mixer, cream together sugar, butter, and eggs. Combine the top 8 dry ingredients. Add to the cream mixture. Add the nuts and mix in well. Remove 1½ cup of the mixture and save for topping.

Press the remaining mixture into an 8-inch square baking pan. Spread jam to within ½ inch from the edge.

Add oats to the reserved mixture and crumble over the preserves. Bake for 40 minutes.

Nutrition:

Calories: 265

Fat: 12.5g

Fiber: 6.1g

Carbs: 28.5g

Protein: 5.9 g

88. Haystacks

Ingredients:

Dairy-free/ Vegetarian-friendly

- √ Haystack Dough
- √ 13⁄4 cups granulated sugar
- √ 1⁄2 cup almond milk
- √ 1⁄4 cup coconut oil
- √ 1⁄4 cup cocoa powder
- √ Other Ingredients
- √ 2 cups gluten-free oats
- √ 1⁄2 cup sunflower seed butter
- √ teaspoon vanilla extract

Preparation Time: 15 minutes

Cooking Time: 0 mins

Servings: 12

Difficulty: Easy

Directions:

Line 2 baking sheets with parchment paper. In a saucepan, all haystack dough must be combined, stir until the mixture comes to a boil for exactly 11⁄2 minutes, Remove the pan from the heat.

Stir in the other ingredients. The batter must then be scooped into the baking sheets by tablespoonfuls and refrigerate until the cookies are hardened.

Nutrition:

Calories: 174

Fat: 4.9g

Fiber: 2.9g

Carbs: 21.5g

Protein: 2.1 g

89. Pecan Pie Bars

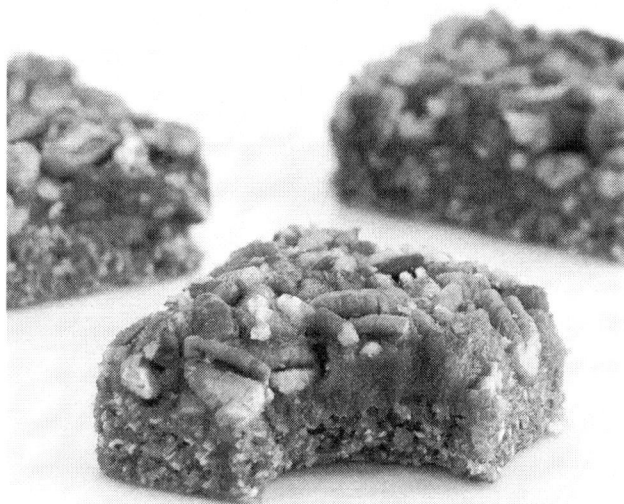

Ingredients:

- √ 1 cup of almonds
- √ 1½ cups pecans
- √ ⅛ tsp. salt
- √ ½ tsp. vanilla extract
- √ 8-oz. dates

Dairy-free/ Vegan

Preparation Time: 15 minutes

Cooking Time: 0 minutes

Servings: 10

Difficulty: Easy

Directions:

Pulse all ingredients in a food processor until combined.

Press into a parchment paper-lined 8 x 8 baking dish. Cover and put in the freezer for 2 hours before cutting into bars.

Nutrition:

Calories: 186

Fat: 8.5g

Fiber: 4.1g

Carbs: 18.5g

Protein: 2.1g

90. Almond Blondies

Ingredients:

Dry:

- √ 1 1/2 cups almond flour
- √ 1/4 cup shredded coconut
- √ 1/2 teaspoon baking soda
- √ 1/4 teaspoon salt

Wet:

- √ 1/4 cup coconut oil
- √ 1/4 cup honey
- √ large egg
- √ 1 teaspoon vanilla extract

Other ingredients:

- √ 1/4 cup walnut
- √ ¼ cup chocolate chips

Dairy-free

Preparation Time: 15 minutes

Cooking Time: 25 minutes

Servings: 9

Difficulty: Easy

Directions: Oven: 325°F.

In a bowl or container, all dry ingredients must be mixed. Set aside. In another bowl or container, combine all the wet ingredients

The dry and wet ingredients must be combined until well blended. Fold in chocolate and walnut pieces. Pour the batter to your baking dish. Bake for 20–25 minutes

Nutrition:

Calories: 199

Fat: 14.5g

Fiber: 4.1g

Carbs: 21.1g

Protein: 2g

91. Energy Bars

Ingredients:

Dry:

- √ 2 cups gluten-free oats
- √ 1¼ cups gluten-free flour
- √ ¾ cup coconut sugar
- √ ¼ cup flaxseed meal
- √ ½ cup almond
- √ ½ cup dried cranberries
- √ ¼ cup pumpkin seeds
- √ ¾ teaspoon cinnamon
- √ ¾ teaspoon salt

Wet:

- √ egg
- √ ½ cup coconut oil
- √ ½ cup honey
- √ teaspoons vanilla extract
- √ ½ cup chocolate chips

Dairy-free/ Vegetarian-friendly

Preparation Time: 15 minutes

Cooking Time: 25 minutes

Servings: 16

Difficulty: Easy

Directions: Oven: 350°F.

In a bowl or container, combine all dry ingredients. Make a well in the center and add then wet ingredients. Mix well using a large spoon or your hands. Add the chocolate chips and combine.

Utilizing your hands, the mixture must be evenly pressed into the prepared pan. Bake until golden brown, about 25 minutes.

Nutrition:

Calories: 181

Fat: 2.5g

Fiber: 10.5g

Carbs: 21.7g

Protein: 9.1g

92. Mixed Fruit Bars

Ingredients:

Dry:

- √ 1¼ cups gluten-free flour
- √ 1¼ cups gluten-free oats
- √ ½ teaspoon baking soda
- √ ¼ teaspoon salt
- √ cup brown sugar

Wet:

- √ ½ cup coconut oil
- √ ¼ cup coconut milk
- √ teaspoon vanilla extract
- √ Other ingredients:
- √ ½ cup slivered almonds
- √ 8 ounces fruit jam

Dairy-free/ Vegan

Preparation Time: 15 minutes

Cooking Time: 30 minutes
Servings: 9
Difficulty: Medium

Directions: Oven: 350°F.

In a bowl or container, combine all the dry ingredients.

In another bowl or container, stir together all the wet ingredients.Combine the two mixture, Press two-thirds of the mixture in the bottom of the prepared pan. Stir the almonds into the remaining mixture and set aside. Bake until golden brown, about 15 minutes.

Take the bars out of the oven and spread with the jam. Sprinkle with the reserved almond-oat mixture. Bake until the crumbs are golden brown, 10 to 15 minutes.

Nutrition:

Calories: 179

Fat: 4.5g

Fiber: 15g

Carbs: 22g

Protein: 10.7g

93. Mississippi Mud Bars

Ingredients:

PEANUT BUTTER CRUST

- √ 2 cups peanut butter
- √ 1½ brown sugar
- √ 1½ cups powdered sugar
- √ 6 tablespoons coconut oil

TOPPING

- √ 3¼ cups chocolate chips
- √ 1½ cups gluten-free mini marshmallows
- √ ½ cup chopped pecans
- √ Salt

Vegetarian-Friendly

Preparation Time: 20 minutes

Cooking Time: 0 minutes

Servings: 12

Difficulty: Easy

Directions:

Crust: Combine all ingredients. Press evenly into the bottom of the pan.

Topping:Microwave the chocolate chips on high in 30-second increments, stirring in between, until melted. Pour half the melted chocolate over the peanut butter crust and spread evenly.

Sprinkle the marshmallows and nuts over the melted chocolate layer, then drizzle the remaining melted chocolate on top. Sprinkle with a pinch of salt. Freeze for 1 hr.

Nutrition:

Calories: 190

Fat: 11.1g

Fiber: 4.2g

Carbs: 22.5g

Protein: 3.1g

94. Fudgy Brownies

Ingredients:

Vegetarian-friendly

- √ ½ cup coconut oil
- √ ½ cup applesauce
- √ 2 cups brown sugar
- √ 1 tsp vanilla
- √ 2 eggs
- √ ¾ cup of cocoa
- √ 1½ cups Gluten-Free Flour
- √ tsp baking powder
- √ ½ tsp salt
- √ ½ cup chopped walnuts

Preparation Time: 25 minutes

Cooking Time: 30 minutes

Servings: 12

Difficulty: Medium

Directions: Oven: 350°F

In a bowl or container, all the ingredients will be mixed. The batter must be spread in a greased 9" x 13" baking pan. Bake for 25—30 minutes.

Nutrition:

Calories: 201

Fat: 11.1g

Fiber: 4.4g

Carbs: 31.7g

Protein: 3.1g

95. Pina Colada Bars

Ingredients:

Dairy-free/ Vegetarian-friendly

Crust:

- √ 1 cup almond meal
- √ 2 tablespoons coconut oil
- √ 1 tablespoon water
- √ tablespoon canola oil

Preparation Time: 35 minutes

Cooking Time: 35 minutes

Servings: 16

Difficulty: Medium

- √ tablespoons sugar
- √ tablespoons coconut flour
- √ ½ teaspoon ground ginger

Filling:

- √ ½ cup of white sugar
- √ cup cottage cheese
- √ 1 ½ tablespoon lemon zest
- √ ¼ cupcream cheese
- √ tablespoon pineapple juice½ teaspoon vanilla extract
- √ 1 egg
- √ Salt

Topping:

- √ cup of chopped pineapple
- √ ¼ cup unsweetened coconut flakes

Directions: Oven: 325°F

Combine all ingredients for the crust then press into the bottom of an 8" greased baking pan. Let the crust bake for 10 minutes.

Filling: Blend all the filling ingredients in a food processor. Spread this over the cooled crust and bake for 35 minutes. Refrigerate until completely chilled. Top with coconut and pineapple.

Nutrition:

Calories: 190

Fat: 5.9g

Fiber: 4.1g

Carbs: 18.7g

Protein: 1.2g

96. Walnut Brownies

Ingredients:

- √ 11/2 cups sugar

Dairy-free

Preparation Time: 15 minutes

- √ 1⁄2 cup Shortening
- √ 2 large eggs
- √ 2 teaspoons vanilla extract
- √ cup self-rising gluten-free flour
- √ 1⁄2 cup cocoa
- √ 1⁄2 cup chopped walnuts

Cooking Time: 25 minutes

Servings: 8

Difficulty: Easy

Directions: Oven: 350° F . An 8" × 8" baking pan must be lined with parchment paper.

In a bowl or container, combine all ingredients except walnuts. Transfer to the baking pan. Sprinkle walnuts on top. Let the brownies bake for about 18–25 minutes.

Nutrition:

Calories: 181

Fat: 8.5g

Fiber: 3.1g

Carbs: 18.7g

Protein: 2.1g

97. Lemon Squares

Ingredients:

CRUST

- √ 13⁄4 cups almond flour
- √ 3 tablespoons shortening
- √ 1 teaspoon coconut flour
- √ 1⁄4 teaspoon baking soda
- √ 1⁄8 teaspoon salt
- √ 2 tablespoons honey
- √ 1⁄4 teaspoon vanilla extract

LEMON CURD FILLING

- √ 6 egg yolks
- √ 1⁄2 cup honey

Dairy-free

Preparation Time: 20 minutes

Cooking Time: 20 minutes

Servings: 9

Difficulty: Medium

- √ teaspoon lemon zest
- √ 1/2 cup lemon juice
- √ 1/4 teaspoon vanilla extract
- √ 6 tablespoons shortening
- √ (Optional) coconut flakes

Directions:

Oven: 315°F. The sides and bottom of an 8" × 8" baking dish must be lightly coated with oil.

For the Crust: Place all dry ingredients in a food processor and place into the prepared baking dish. Now, the dough must be evenly pressed into the bottom part of the dish. Bake the crust for 8–10 minutes.

For the Lemon Curd Filling: In a small saucepan, whisk all listed ingredients and heat until slightly thickened. Cool down. Once cool, put in the lemon curd to the cooled crust/Bake at 315°F for approximately 20 minutes.

For a decorative touch, sprinkle the bars with unsweetened shredded coconut, if desired.

Nutrition:

Calories: 201

Fat: 12g

Fiber: 5g

Carbs: 22.5g

Protein: 1.2g

98. Autumn Pumpkin Bars

Ingredients:

PUMPKIN BARS

- √ 1 cup almond flour
- √ 1 teaspoon coconut flour
- √ 1/2 teaspoon baking soda
- √ 1/4 teaspoon sea salt
- √ 1/2 cup pumpkin purée

Dairy-free

Preparation Time: 35 minutes

Cooking Time: 25 minutes

Servings: 9

Difficulty: Medium

- √ 1/3 cup honey
- √ 2 large eggs
- √ 11/2 teaspoons Pumpkin Pie Spice
- √ 1/4 teaspoon vanilla extract

PRALINE TOPPING

- √ tablespoon coconut oil
- √ teaspoons honey
- √ 1/8 teaspoon ground cinnamon
- √ 1/3 cup pecan pieces

Directions: Oven: 350°F . Lightly oil an 8" × 8" baking dish; set aside.

In a bowl or container, put in all pumplom bar ingredients and mix until well combined. Then spoon the batter into the prepared baking dish.

Praline Topping: In a bowl or container, add all praling topping.

Top the praline topping evenly across the top of the pumpkin bar batter, making sure to press it into the batter a bit gently. Let it bake for around 25 minutes.

Nutrition:

Calories: 187

Fat: 12g

Fiber: 4.1g

Carbs: 22g

Protein: 1.1g

99. Pumpkin Bars

Ingredients:

CRUST

- √ 130 grams gluten-free graham crumbs
- √ 60 grams pumpkin seeds

Dairy-free

Preparation Time: 20 minutes

Cooking Time: 45 minutes

Servings: 16

√ 2 tablespoons granulated sugar

√ 8 tablespoons coconut oil

FILLING

√ 32 grams of Almond flour

√ 1½ teaspoons pumpkin pie spice

√ teaspoon cinnamon

√ ¼ teaspoon xanthan gum

√ ¼ teaspoon salt

√ 1 (8-ounce) vegan cream cheese

√ 1 (15-ounce) can pumpkin puree

√ 200 grams brown sugar

√ 2 eggs

√ 1¼ cups coconut milk

√ 2 teaspoons vanilla extract

Directions: Oven: 350°F. A 9-by-9-inch baking pan must be lined with parchment paper.

In a food processor, all crust ingredients must be pulsed. The crust mixture must be pressed firmly into the bottom of the prepared pan.Bake for 8 minutes. In a small bowl, all filling ingredients must be whisked until smooth. The filling will be poured into the crust. Let it bake for about 40-50 minutes.

Nutrition:

Calories: 179

Fat: 9.7g

Fiber: 7.5g

Carbs: 22.7g

Protein: 2.7g

100. Apple Blondies

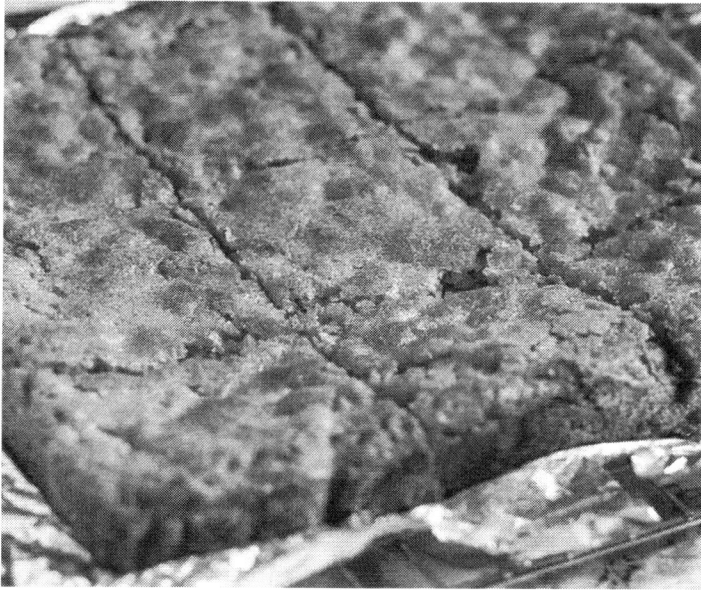

Ingredients:

FILLING

- √ 1 tablespoon coconut oil
- √ 2 cups apples
- √ 2 tablespoons brown sugar
- √ teaspoon cinnamon
- √ 1 teaspoon vanilla extract

BLONDIE

- √ ½ cup coconut oil
- √ ¾ cup brown sugar
- √ 2 large eggs
- √ tablespoon vanilla extract
- √ 1½ cups gluten-free flour
- √ 1 teaspoon baking powder
- √ 1 teaspoon cinnamon
- √ ⅛ teaspoon nutmeg
- √ ½ teaspoon salt

Vegetarian-friendly

Preparation Time: 25 minutes

Cooking Time: 45 minutes

Servings: 9

Difficulty: Medium

GLAZE

- √   cup confectioners' sugar
- √   tablespoons maple syrup
- √   1 teaspoon vanilla extract

Directions:

Oven: 350F. Line an 8" × 8" baking pan with parchment paper and coat with gluten-free nonstick cooking spray.

In a small saucepan, combine all filling ingredients and cook for 5 minutes. In a bowl or container, beat all blondie ingredients. Pour batter into prepared pan. Pour apple filling on top of blondie batter and spread to cover evenly. Bake for 35–45 minutes until golden brown.

In a small bowl, stir together the glaze ingredients until smooth. Drizzle glaze on top of warm blondies.

Nutrition:

Calories: 190

Fat: 11.5g

Fiber: 4.1g

Carbs: 21.8g

Protein: 1.3g

---

101.   **No-Bake Brownie Bites**

Ingredients:

Dairy-free/ Vegan

- √   ½ cup dates
- √   ⅓ cup sunflower seed butter
- √   ⅓ cup cocoa power
- √   2 teaspoons vanilla extract
- √   ¼ teaspoon salt

Preparation Time: 15 minutes

Cooking Time: 0 minutes

Servings: 12

Difficulty: Easy

Topping:

- √   2 tablespoons chocolate chips

Directions:

Combine all ingredients in a food processor. Spoon the mixture into an 8-by-5-inch glass dish.

It must be topped with chocolate chips and press them into the brownies a bit.

Nutrition:

Calories: 144

Fat: 5g

Fiber: 2.5g

Carbs: 15.4g

Protein: 2g

Chapter 8. <u>CANDY AND CONFECTIONS</u>

102.   Coconut Bonbons

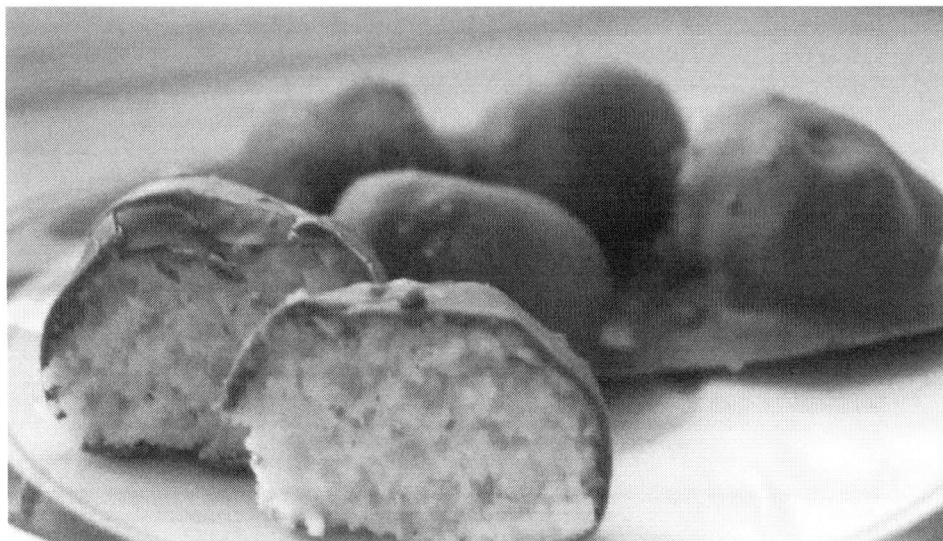

Ingredients:

Bonbon:

- √ 2 2/3 cups sweetened flaked coconut
- √ 1/4 cup coconut milk
- √ 2 tablespoons coconut oil
- √ tablespoon agave
- √ 1/2 teaspoon vanilla extract
- √ 1/4 teaspoon salt

For dipping:

- √ 1/2 cup chocolate chips, melted and cooled

Dairy-free/ Vegan

Preparation Time: 45 minutes

Cooking Time: 5 minutes

Servings: 12

Difficulty: Easy

Directions:

Line a baking sheet with parchment paper. In a bowl or container, stir together all bonbon ingredients drop dough by tablespoonfuls, roll into balls into the sheet and freeze for 1hr.

After, dip the bottoms into the cooled melted chocolate. Return the bonbons to the freezer for at least 20 minutes.

Nutrition:

Calories: 154

Fat: 7.4g

Fiber: 2.3g

Carbs: 15.7g

Protein: 1.4g

103.   Dark Chocolate Fudge

Dairy-free/ Vegan

Preparation Time: 15 minutes

Cooking Time: 0 minutes

Servings: 16

Difficulty: Easy

Ingredients:

- √ 33⁄4 cups cocoa powder
- √ 3 cups agave
- √ 11⁄2 cups coconut oil
- √ 3⁄4 teaspoon espresso powder
- √ 1⁄2 teaspoon salt

Dairy-free/ Vegan

Preparation Time: 15 minutes

Cooking Time: 0 minutes

Servings: 16

Difficulty: Easy

Directions:

An 8-inch square baking pan must be greased with a little canola oil. In a bowl or container, stir together all the ingredients. Spread into the prepared pan and freeze for 2 hours.

Nutrition:

Calories: 151

Fat:6.5g

Fiber: 2.5g

Carbs: 14.3g

Protein: 1.9g

104.   Choconut Butter Balls

Ingredients:

For balls:

- √ 1¼ cups peanut butter
- √ 1 lb. bag powdered sugar
- √ ½ cup of coconut oil
- √ For dipping:
- √ 2 cups chocolate chips

Vegetarian-friendly

Preparation Time: 20 minutes

Cooking Time: 0 mins

Servings: 25

Difficulty: Easy

Directions:

Mix all peanut butter ball ingredients.Roll into bite-sized balls and place them on a cookie sheet. Put a toothpick in each ball and refrigerate for 2 hours. Microwave chocolate chips until it's melted.
Dip chilled balls one by one into the chocolate. Refrigerate until served.

Nutrition:

Calories: 149

Fat: 2.5g

Fiber: 1.5g

Carbs: 18.7g

Protein: 1.7g

105.   Double Chocolate Bites

Ingredients:

- √ 10 dates
- √ 4 tablespoons pumpkin seeds
- √ 2 tablespoons cocoa powder
- √ 4 tablespoons chocolate chips, divided
- √ 2 teaspoons vanilla extract

Dairy-free/ Vegan

Preparation Time: 15 minutes

Cooking Time: 0 minutes

Servings: 6

Difficulty: Easy

Directions:

Pulse or blend all ingredients except half of the chocolate chips.Roll into balls the dip the bottoms of each in the remaining melted chocolate chips. Chill them for 30 minutes.

Nutrition:

Calories: 167

Fat: 5.5g

Fiber: 3.1g

Carbs: 14.7g

Protein: 2g

106.   Orange Macaroons

Ingredients:

Dairy-free/ Vegetarian-friendly

√   1 egg

√   2½ tablespoons sugar

√   1 cup coconut flakes

√   ½ teaspoon vanilla extract

√   2 tablespoons cornstarch

√   ⅛ teaspoon salt

√   2 teaspoons orange zest

Preparation Time: 10 minutes

Cooking Time: 10 minutes

Servings: 10

Difficulty: Medium

Directions: Oven: 350°F. Line a baking sheet with parchment paper.

In a bowl or container, all the ingredients must be combined. Scoop level 1-tablespoon measures of batter onto the baking sheet. Bake for about 9 minutes.

Nutrition:

Calories: 165

Fat: 11.5g

Fiber: 8.5g

Carbs: 22.1g

Protein: 1.2g

107. Chocolate Truffles

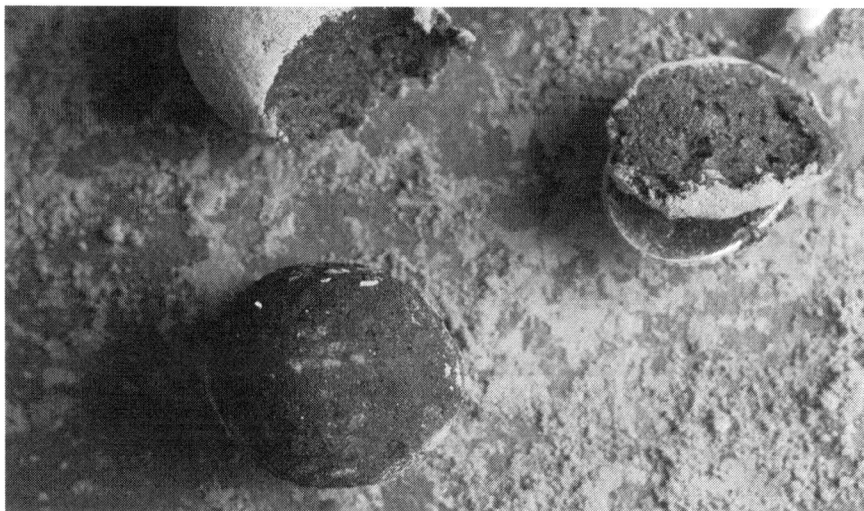

Ingredients:

TRUFFLES:

- √ 1 cup cashews
- √ 1 cup dates
- √ 1 cup of water
- √ ½ cup of coconut milk powder
- √ ½ cup cocoa powder
- √ ¼ cup coconut flour
- √ teaspoon vanilla extract

COATING:

- √ 3 tablespoons confectioners' sugar
- √ 3 tablespoons cocoa powder

Dairy-free/ Vegan

Preparation Time: 40 minutes

Cooking Time: 0 minutes
Servings: 12
Difficulty: Medium

Directions:

Truffles: Soak the cashews and dates in the water for 1 hour. Drain the cashews and dates, transfer to a food processor, and pulse until smooth. In a bowl or container, stir remaining ingredients. Stir in the cashew and date mixture until combined. Chill for 30 minutes. Roll the truffle mixture into 12 balls and place on the baking sheet and freeze for an hr.

Coating: In a bowl or container, stir together all ingredients. Roll truffles in the coating.

Nutrition:

Calories: 158

Fat: 5.4g

Fiber: 3.1g

Carbs: 19.7g

Protein: 1.3g

108.   Fudge Pops

Ingredients:

- √ 1 can coconut milk, divided
- √ 1½ teaspoons agar-agar
- √ ½ cup honey
- √ ⅓ cup cocoa powder
- √ 2 teaspoons vanilla extract

Dairy-free/ Vegan

Preparation Time: 10 minutes
Cooking Time: 5 minutes
Servings: 5
Difficulty: Easy

Directions:

Pour ½ cup of the coconut milk into a small saucepan and sprinkle with the gelatin. Bring to a boil and boil for 2 minutes.Set aside to cool slightly. In a blender, put in the gelatin plus the remaining ingredients. Pour into the molds. Freeze for 4 hours.

Nutrition:

Calories: 141

Fat: 6.1g

Fiber: 3.2g

Carbs: 14.7g

Protein: 1.1g

109.   Matcha Macaroons

Ingredients:

- √ 3 cups coconut flakes
- √ 4 egg whites

Dairy-free/ Vegetarian-friendly

Preparation Time: 25 minutes
Cooking Time: 15 minutes

- √ ¾ cup granulated sugar
- √ ½ cup almond meal
- √ tablespoon matcha powder
- √ 1 teaspoon vanilla extract
- √ ¼ teaspoon salt

Servings: 24
Difficulty: Easy

Directions: Oven: 350°F.

Place the coconut on a baking sheet and bake until toasted. In a bowl or container, beat all remaining ingredients. Stir in the toasted coconut/

Roll the dough into 1½-inch balls and put in the sheet. Bake until golden brown, 15 minutes.

Nutrition:

Calories: 147

Fat: 5.4g

Fiber: 3.1g

Carbs: 13.6g

Protein: 1.2g

110.   **Classic Coconut Macaroons**

Ingredients:

Dairy-free/ Vegetarian-friendly

- √ 42 grams of almond flour
- √ ¼ teaspoon xanthan gum
- √ ¼ teaspoon salt
- √ 1 can coconut milk
- √ ½ teaspoon almond extract
- √ teaspoon vanilla extract
- √ 1 egg white
- √ 100 grams coconut flakes

Preparation Time: 45 minutes
Cooking Time: 15 minutes
Servings: 12
Difficulty: Easy

Directions: Oven: 350°F

In a container or bowl, whisk the flour, xanthan gum, and salt to combine. In another container, add all other ingredients. Combine the two and chill for 30 mins. Scoop the macaroons onto the baking sheets. Let the macaroons bake for 15 minutes.

Nutrition:

Calories: 143

Fat: 8.3g

Fiber: 3.3g

Carbs: 16.4g

Protein: 2.4g

111.   Southern Pralines

Ingredients:

- √ 1 cup brown sugar
- √ 1 cup white sugar
- √ ½ cup heavy cream
- √ 2 tablespoons coconut oil

Preparation Time: 10 minutes

Cooking Time: 25 minutes

Servings: 24

Difficulty: Easy

Other ingredients

- √ cup pecans
- √ 1 teaspoon vanilla extract
- √ Salt

Directions:

In a heated saucepan, stir and cook the first four ingredients. It must reach the "softball" stage (238 to 240°F on a candy thermometer). Immediately remove from the heat. Add the pecans and vanilla. Stir together. Working quickly, drop large spoonful 2 inches apart onto the parchment paper. Garnish with salt.

Nutrition:

Calories: 161

Fat: 5.9g

Fiber: 2.1g

Carbs: 18.6g

Protein: 1.6g

112.   Chocolate Covered Macaroons

Ingredients: *Dairy-free/ Vegetarian-friendly*

- √   3 egg whites
- √   ¼ teaspoon cream of tartar
- √   ⅛ teaspoon salt
- √   ¼ teaspoon almond extract
- √   ½ cup granulated sugar
- √   ⅔ cup gluten-free flour with xanthan gum
- √   4 cups coconut flakes
- √   1½ cups chocolate chips
- √   2 teaspoons coconut oil

Preparation Time: 40 minutes

Cooking Time: 20 minutes

Servings: 20

Difficulty: Medium

Directions: Oven: 350°F

In a bowl or container, beat egg whites, cream of tartar, and salt until foamy. Add almond extract, sugar, flour and continue to beat until stiff. Stir in shredded coconut.

Scoop out dough using a cookie scoop and place on baking sheets. Bake for 18–20 minutes.

In a microwave-safe dish, melt chocolate chips and add coconut oil and stir. Dip the top of each cookie into the melted chocolate.

Nutrition:

Calories: 143

Fat: 7.6g

Fiber: 1.4g

Carbs: 16.6g

Protein: 2.9g

113.   Butter Cups

Ingredients: *Dairy-free/ Vegan*

COATING

- √   1½ cups chocolate chips
- √   2 teaspoons coconut oil

Preparation Time: 30 minutes

Cooking Time: 1 minute

Servings: 12

FILLING

- √ ¼ cup sunflower seed butter
- √ tablespoon maple syrup
- √ ½ tablespoon coconut flour
- √ ¼ teaspoon salt

Directions:

Line a 12-cup mini muffin tin with parchment liners to prevent sticking. Set aside. To make the coating, melt the chocolate and oil in a double boiler. Into each paper liner, spoon about 2 teaspoons of the melted chocolate coating. Tap the pan to settle the chocolate. Refrigerate the tin for 10 minutes to allow the chocolate to set.

In a bowl or container, combine filling ingredients. Scoop out 1-teaspoon portions of the filling and form into balls. Remove the muffin tin from the refrigerator. Gently press each ball of filling to flatten it into a disk. Place each disk of filling on top of each chocolate cup. Top each disk of filling with about 1½ teaspoons of melted chocolate. Refrigerate for 30 minutes.

Nutrition:

Calories: 149

Fat: 8.7g

Fiber: 3.5g

Carbs: 19.9g

Protein: 1.3 g

114. Almond Meringue

Ingredients:

Dairy-free/ Vegetarian-friendly

- √ 4 egg whites
- √ ¼ teaspoon cream of tartar
- √ ½ cup powdered sugar
- √ 1 teaspoon almond extract

Preparation Time: 30 minutes

Cooking Time: 60 minutes

Servings: 12

Difficulty: Medium

Directions:

Oven: 225°F . Line a 9x13-inch baking sheet (not nonstick) with parchment paper.

In a bowl or container, beat the egg whites on low speed until foamy. Add the cream of tartar and beat on medium speed until soft peaks form. Add the powdered sugar gradually— 2 tablespoons at a time— while beating to very stiff peaks. Stir in the almond extract.

Transfer the batter to a piping bag and pipe 24 rounds, leaving 1 inch between cookies.

Bake until the cookies are firm and crisp, about 2 hours, turning the baking sheet 180 degrees after 1 hour to assure even baking.

Nutrition:

Calories: 161

Fat: 8.9g

Fiber: 2.1g

Carbs: 17.7g

Protein: 1.4g

Chapter 9. <u>PUDDING AND SPOON DESSERTS</u>

115.   Banana Quinoa Pudding

Ingredients:

Dairy-free/ Vegan

- √ 1 cup quinoa
- √ 2 cups of water
- √ 3 ripe bananas
- √ 4 cups of water
- √ 4 tbsp sugar
- √ tsp vanilla extract

Preparation Time: 15 minutes

Cooking Time: 25 minutes

Servings: 4

Difficulty: Easy

Directions:

Wash and cook quinoa according to package directions. In a separate bowl, blend sugar and bananas until smooth. Add to the quinoa. Heat over medium heat, stirring until creamy. Stir in vanilla and serve warm.

Nutrition:

Calories: 241

Fat: 3.5g

Fiber: 4.2g

Carbs: 42 g

Protein: 7.2g

116.   Chocolate Pots De Crème

Ingredients:

Dairy-free/ Vegan

- √ 2 very ripe avocados
- √ 3/4 cup cocoa powder
- √ 2/3 cup maple syrup
- √ 1/4 cup agave syrup
- √ teaspoon vanilla extract
- √ 1/2 teaspoon espresso powder
- √ 1/2 teaspoon salt

Preparation Time: 15 minutes

Cooking Time: 0 minutes

Servings: 6

Difficulty: Easy

Directions:

Blend all ingredients and pour the pudding intoramekins. Chill, and serve.

Nutrition:

Calories: 201

Fat: 15g

Fiber: 5.4g

Carbs: 29g

Protein: 4.3g

---

117.   Chocolate Date Pudding

Ingredients:

- √ 2 avocados
- √ 1/2 cup dates
- √ 1/2 cup water
- √ 5 tablespoons cacao powder
- √ 2 teaspoons vanilla extract
- √ Salt

Dairy-free/ Vegan

Preparation Time: 10 minutes

Cooking Time: 0 minutes

Servings: 4

Difficulty: Easy

Directions:

Blend all ingredients until smooth. Pour into glasses.

Refrigerate for a few hours to let the pudding set.

Nutrition:

Calories: 221

Fat: 11.9g

Fiber: 5.4g

Carbs: 29.5g

Protein: 1.8g

118.   Mango Coconut Pudding

Ingredients:

Dairy-free/ Vegan

- √ 1 cup cashew nuts, soaked
- √ 1 cup coconut meat
- √ 1/2 cup water
- √ 4 tablespoons honey
- √ tablespoon lemon juice
- √ 1 teaspoon vanilla extract
- √ tablespoons lecithin
- √ tablespoons coconut oil

Preparation Time: 20 minutes

Cooking Time: 0 minutes

Servings: 5

Difficulty: Easy

Garnish:

- √ mango, sliced

Directions:

All the ingredients must be blended except for the coconut oil and lecithin. Blend until smooth. Add lecithin and coconut oil and blend until well incorporated. Pour into glasses. Decorate with sliced mango. Refrigerate for a few hours to let the pudding set.

Nutrition:

Calories: 198

Fat: 13.9g

Fiber: 7.9g

Carbs: 31g

Protein: 5.4g

119.   Cherry Apple Coconut Rice Pudding

Ingredients:

Dairy-free/ Vegan

- √ 1 cup Arborio rice
- √ 15-ounce coconut milk
- √ 1 cup cherries
- √ 1 cup applesauce

Preparation Time: 5 minutes

Cooking Time: 60 minutes

Servings: 4

Difficulty: Easy

Directions: Oven: 325°F

Rinse rice. All listed ingredients will be combined and placed in a covered casserole. Bake 1 hour until the rice has absorbed most of the liquid.

Nutrition:

Calories: 224

Fat: 12.9g

Fiber: 5.4g

Carbs: 29.5g

Protein: 5.4g

120. Pineapple Coconut Rice Pudding

Ingredients:

- √ 1 (15-ounce) can coconut milk
- √ 1 (15-ounce) can crushed pineapple
- √ 1 cup Arborio rice

Dairy-free/ Vegan

Preparation Time: 15 minutes

Cooking Time: 60 minutes

Servings: 8

Directions: Oven: 325°F

Difficulty: Easy

In a saucepan, let crushed pineapple with juice and coconut milk to a boil.

Rinse rice with cold water through a colander. Combine rice with heated coconut milk and pineapple mixture and pour it into a casserole dish. Cover dish with aluminum foil. Bake 1 hour until the rice has absorbed most of the liquid but is still creamy.

Nutrition:

Calories: 221

Fat: 15g

Fiber: 6.1g

Carbs: 29.9g

Protein: 1.2g

121. Vanilla Rice Pudding

Ingredients:

- √ 1 cup Arborio rice

Dairy-free/ Vegan

Preparation Time: 15 minutes

- √ 4 cups almond milk
- √ 1/2 cup maple syrup
- √ 2 tablespoons vanilla extract

Cooking Time: 60 minutes

Servings: 8

Difficulty: Easy

Directions:

Preheat oven to 325°F. Rinse rice.

In a small saucepan, bring other ingredients to a boil. Combine liquid and rice in a casserole dish.

Bake 1 hour until most of the liquid has been absorbed by the rice but still creamy.

Nutrition:

Calories: 233

Fat: 18.5g

Fiber: 1.4g

Carbs: 35.4g

Protein: 2g

122.   Key Lime Parfait

Ingredients:

Dairy-free/ Vegan

- √ ½ cup lime juice
- √ 1 can condensed milk
- √ 9-ounce whipped topping
- √ ½ cup gluten-free graham crumbs, divided

Preparation Time: 15 minutes

Cooking Time: 0 minutes

Servings: 4

Difficulty: easy

Directions:

In a bowl or container, the first three ingredients must be combined.Divide half the mixture evenly between 4 dessert dishes. Top each with graham crumbs. Add the remaining filling, then sprinkle graham crumbs on top of each serving.

Chill for at least 2 hours. Garnish each serving with 1 tablespoon of additional whipped topping.

Nutrition:

Calories: 214

Fat: 5.6g

Fiber: 9.5g

Carbs: 23.8g

Protein: 1.2g

123.   Chocolate Mousse

Ingredients:

Dairy-free/ Vegan

√ 1 cup chocolate chips

√ 1 can coconut milk

√ 2 tablespoons pure maple syrup

√ ½ tablespoon vanilla extract

√ ⅛ teaspoon salt

Preparation Time: 15 minutes

Cooking Time: 0 minutes

Servings: 6

Difficulty: Easy

Directions:

Melt the chocolate chips in the microwave. Whisk all the other ingredients with the melted chocolate. Pour the mixture into dessert bowls. Chill until the mousse is set.

Nutrition:

Calories: 231

Fat: 18.4g

Fiber: 3.3g

Carbs: 18.6g

Protein: 2.5g

124.   Chia Pudding

Ingredients:

Dairy-free/ Vegan

√ 2 cups almond milk

√ ⅔ cup chia seeds

√ 2 tablespoons maple syrup

√ 1 teaspoon vanilla extract

√ Garnish

√ Sliced pears

√ Cacao nibs

Preparation Time: 5 minutes

Cooking Time: 25 minutes

Servings: 4

Difficulty: Easy

Directions:

In a bowl or container, whisk all ingredients except the garnish. Cover and refrigerate for 25 minutes. Serve with sliced pears and cacao nibs.

Nutrition:

Calories: 143

Fat: 2.8g

Fiber: 6.5g

Carbs: 11.7g

Protein: 4.3g

125. Chocolate Souffle

Ingredients:

√ ½ cup chocolate chips
√ 3 tablespoons coconut oil
√ 1 cup almond flour
√ ¼ cup arrowroot starch
√ ¼ cup of coconut sugar
√ ¼ cup cocoa powder
√ ¼ teaspoon of salt
√ ½ teaspoon baking powder
√ ½ cup coconut milk
√ ¼ cup maple syrup
√ ½ teaspoon vinegar
√ ½ teaspoon vanilla extract

Dairy-free/ Vegan

Preparation Time: 10 minutes
Cooking Time: 20 minutes
Servings: 2
Difficulty: Hard

Directions: Oven: 325°F Spray two ramekins with cooking spray.

In a saucepan, melt the chocolate chips and coconut oil. Remove from the heat and set aside. In a bowl or container, mix the dry ingredients.

In another bowl or container, whisk together the other wet ingredients. Combine in the melted chocolate mixture and dry mixture. The batter must be distributed between the ramekins. Bake for 15 minutes.

Nutrition:

Calories: 254

Fat: 11.5g

Fiber: 4.1g

Carbs: 29.7g

Protein: 1.4g

126.   Old-Fashion Rice Pudding

Ingredients:

Vegetarian-friendly

- √   3⁄4 cup long-grain rice
- √   3 cups almond milk
- √   3⁄4 cup granulated sugar
- √   3⁄4 teaspoon cinnamon
- √   Salt
- √   1⁄3 cup coconut oil

Preparation Time: 15 minutes

Cooking Time: 3 hrs.

Servings: 6

Difficulty: Easy

Directions:

Using a colander, wash the rice under cold water then pour it into a slow cooker. Put in the other listed ingredients and stir. Cover and cook on high for 21/2–3 hours until the rice has absorbed the liquid.

Nutrition:

Calories: 243

Fat: 5.5g

Fiber: 3.9g

Carbs: 31.5g

Protein: 4.3g

127.   Orange Polenta

Ingredients:

Dairy-free/ Vegetarian-friendly

Polenta:

- √   1 ½ cups coconut milk

Preparation Time: 15 minutes

Cooking Time: 10 minutes

- √ 2 cups of water
- √ ¾ cup of instant polenta
- √ ¼ teaspoon salt
- √ Other ingredients:
- √ Zest from orange
- √ ¼ cup cream cheese
- √ ¼ cup Greek yogurt
- √ orange segments

Servings: 2
Difficulty: Easy

Garnish:

- √ 4 tablespoons honey
- √ teaspoon tarragon

Directions:

Mix water, salt, milk and polenta in a saucepan and boil. Remove from heat and mix in the other ingredients. Divide between four bowls. Garnish with the orange pieces and sprinkle with tarragon.

Nutrition:

Calories: 201

Fat: 2.5g

Fiber: 3.1g

Carbs: 19.5g

Protein: 3.1g

128.   **Pumpkin Crème Brulee**

Ingredients:

Dairy-free/ Vegetarian-friendly

- √ 4 cups of almond milk
- √ ¼ teaspoon salt
- √ ¼ teaspoon ground ginger
- √ 1/8 teaspoon cloves
- √ teaspoon cinnamon
- √ teaspoons vanilla extract
- √ ¼ cup brown sugar

Preparation Time: 20 minutes
Cooking Time: 17 minutes
Servings: 12
Difficulty: Medium

- √ 1 cup whte sugar
- √ 1 cup pumpkin puree
- √ 16 eggs yolks

Directions: Oven: 325°F

Using a large, heavy saucepan, combine and whisk all ingredients then pour into ramekins and arrange them on a baking sheet. Bake the crème Brulee for about 15 minutes until set then chill for 6 hrs. Top with a teaspoon of sugar on top and torch.

Nutrition:

Calories: 185

Fat: 5.5g

Fiber: 3.5g

Carbs: 27g

Protein: 4.1g

129.   Pavlova

Ingredients:

Dairy-free/ Vegetarian-friendly

- √ 4 egg whites
- √ 1 teaspoon vinegar
- √ 1/2 cup sugar
- √ 1 cup heavy cream
- √ 3 tablespoons confectioners' sugar
- √ 1/2 teaspoon vanilla
- √ banana, sliced
- √ quart strawberries

Preparation Time: 35 minutes

Cooking Time: 2 hrs.

Servings: 6

Difficulty: Medium

Directions: Oven: 200° F

In a container or bowl, the egg whites must be whisked, and as they stiffen, add the vinegar and slowly add the sugar. Pour into a 9-glass pie pan then bake the meringue for 2 hours.

In a bowl or container, whip the cream and mix in the confectioners' sugar and vanilla.

Sliced layers of banana onto the bottom of the cooled meringue crust. Add a layer of whipped cream. Sprinkle with halved strawberries.

Add one more layer of whipped cream and decorate with the whole strawberries.

Nutrition:

Calories: 191

Fat: 9.5g

Fiber: 3.5g

Carbs: 21.7g

Protein: 4.1g

130.   Rice Pudding with Cherry Sauce

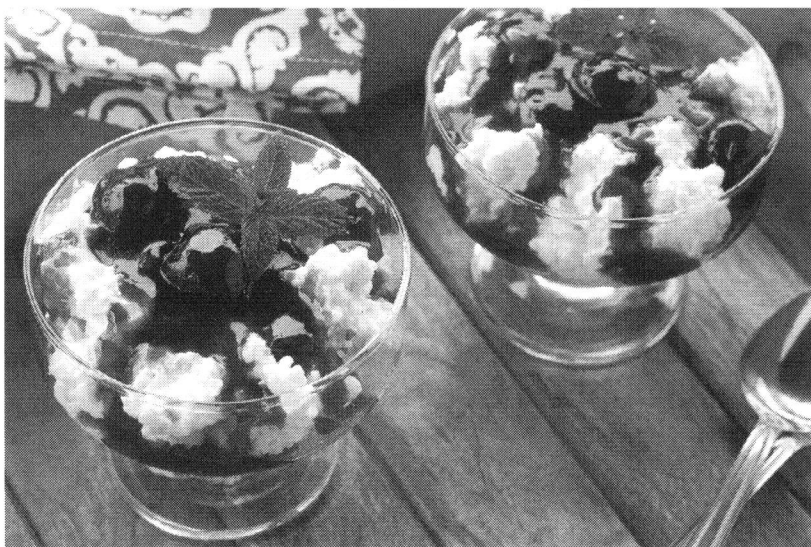

Ingredients:

Cherry sauce:

- √ 1/4 cup water
- √ 1 tablespoon lemon juice
- √ 1 tablespoon sugar
- √ salt
- √ 2 tablespoons cornstarch
- √ 2 cups frozen cherries

Rice cream:

- √ 1/2 cups water

Dairy-free/ Vegetarian-friendly

Preparation Time: 10 minutes

Cooking Time: 40 minutes

Servings: 8

Difficulty: Medium

- √ 1/4 teaspoon salt
- √ 1 cup short-grain white rice
- √ cups of almond milk
- √ 1/4 cup slivered almonds
- √ 1 cup heavy cream
- √ 1/4 cup granulated sugar
- √ 1 teaspoon vanilla extract

Directions:

For the cherry sauce: Combine all ingredients and cook for 5-10 minutes until thick.

For the rice cream: Combine all rice cream ingredients except whippe creamand cook in a pot for 40 minutes. After, stir in the almonds

Whip the cream until it forms soft peaks. Carefully fold in the whipped cream and rice. Scoop individual portions of rice cream.Spoon some cherry sauce over it and serve.

Nutrition:

Calories: 112

Fat: 2.5g

Fiber: 5.5g

Carbs: 21.7g

Protein: 3.7g

131.   Italian Tiramisu

Ingredients:

VANILLA CASHEW CREAM

Dairy-free/ Vegan

Preparation Time: 55 minutes

- √ 2 cups raw whole cashews, soaked in water overnight, drained and rinsed
- √ ½ cup unsweetened almond milk
- √ ¼ cup maple syrup
- √ 1 teaspoon vanilla extract

Cooking Time: 15 minutes

Servings: 12

Difficulty: Medium

COCONUT CREAM

- √ cup coconut cream

√ 1 tablespoon maple syrup

√ ½ teaspoon vanilla extract

SHEET CAKE

√ 2 flax eggs (4 tablespoons water +2 tablespoons ground flaxseed)

√ 2 cups brown rice flour

√ cup almond flour

√ ¾ cup sugar

√ 2 teaspoons baking powder

√ teaspoon baking soda

√ ½ teaspoon of sea salt

√ 1 cup coconut milk

√ ¼ cup maple syrup

√ ¼ cup melted coconut oil

√ teaspoon vanilla extract

FOR THE SAUCE

√ ¾ cup coconut milk

√ ½ cup cocoa powder

√ ½ cup sugar

√ ¼ cup brewed coffee

√ teaspoon vanilla extract

√ ¼ teaspoon of salt

Directions:

In a high-speed blender, blend all cashew cream ingredients until smooth.

To make the coconut whipped cream, use a hand mixer to beat the ingredients until fluffy.

Combine the two mixture and chill. (This is the vegan mascarpone). Oven: 350°F

Line a baking sheet with parchment paper. (I recommend a 15-by-10-inch half sheet pan.)

To make the sheet cake, in another medium bowl, prepare the flax eggs by whisking together the ground flaxseed and water. Set aside for at least 10 minutes.

In a bowl or container, all other ingredients and add in the flax eggs.

Now, the batter must be transferred to the prepared baking sheet Let the meringue cook for about 15 minutes. Once cooled, cut the sheet cake in half and then into 2-by-4-inch rectangles. Lay half of the rectangles on the bottom of a 9-by-13-inch baking dish.

To make the sauce, in a small saucepan over medium-high heat, combine all ingredients and cook for 10 minutes.

Half of the sauce must be poured on top of the cake in the baking dish, spreading evenly with a spatula if needed. Spread half of the vegan mascarpone on top. Layer the remaining sheet cake sections, remaining sauce, and remaining mascarpone. Dust with cocoa powder, if desired.

Nutrition:

Calories: 165

Fat: 5g

Fiber: 3.9g

Carbs: 31.5g

Protein: 2.6g

132.   Southern Banana Pudding

Ingredients:

- √   5-ounce package gluten-free vanilla pudding mix
- √   2 cups of milk
- √   8-ounce cream cheese, softened
- √   14-ounce condensed milk
- √   5 cups Coconut Whipped Cream, divided
- √   6 cups crushed gluten-free graham cracker
- √   cup of sugar
- √   1 cup coconut oil, melted
- √   4 bananas, sliced

Preparation Time: 20 minutes

Cooking Time: 0 minutes

Servings: 12

Difficulty: Easy

Directions:

In a bowl or container, stir the milk and pudding mix together. Add the cream cheese and condensed milk. Whisk until smooth. Add 2 cups of whipped cream and whip until smooth.

In a bowl or container, combine the graham crackers, sugar, and coconut oil and mix well. Half of the mixture will then be spread in the bottom of a 9-by-13-inch baking pan. Lay half the sliced bananas on top of the cookie crust in an even layer, then put in half amount of the vanilla pudding on top of the bananas.   Repeat these three layers once more, ending with the pudding mixture.

Top with the remaining 3 cups of whipped cream and the remaining graham cracker crumbles.

Nutrition:

Calories: 243

Fat: 15.1g

Fiber: 8.5g

Carbs: 22.7g

Protein: 5g

Chapter 10. <u>RUSTIC FRUIT DESSERTS</u>

133. Spiced Baked Apples

Ingredients:

- √ 8 apples

Filling:

- √ 1/3 cup walnuts, crushed
- √ 3/4 cup sugar
- √ 3 tbsp raisins, soaked
- √ Vanilla extract
- √ Cinnamon

Dairy-free/ Vegan

Preparation Time: 20 minutes

Cooking Time: 30 minutes

Servings: 4

Difficulty: Easy

Directions: Oven: 350°F

Peel and carefully hollow the apples. Prepare stuffing by mixing all ingredients. Stuff the apples and place in a dish, pour over 1 tbsp of water, and bake the apples for 30 minutes.

Nutrition:

Calories: 85

Fat: 0.5g

Fiber: 4.5g

Carbs: 23.g

Protein: 0.1 g

134. Nutty Berry Quinoa

Ingredients:

- √ ½ cup quinoa
- √ 1 cup of water
- √ ¼ cup fresh blueberries or raspberries
- √ 1 tbsp walnuts
- √ 3-4 tbsp maple syrup
- √ tbsp chia seeds

Dairy-free/ Vegan

Preparation Time: 15 minutes

Cooking Time: 25 minutes

Servings: 2

Difficulty: Easy

Directions:

Cook quinoa according to package directions. When ready, add walnuts and cinnamon, place a portion of the quinoa into a bowl, and top with fresh blueberries, chia seeds, and maple syrup.

Nutrition:

Calories: 276

Fat: 9.5g

Fiber: 12.5g

Carbs: 42.7g

Protein: 11.7g

135.   Raspberry Almond Parfait

Ingredients:

Dairy-free/ Vegan

Pudding:

- √ 3 tablespoons chia seeds
- √ 1 cup almond milk
- √ 1½ tablespoons honey
- √ ¼ teaspoon cinnamon

Raspberry Sauce:

- √ cup raspberries
- √ ½ tablespoon honey
- √ Lemon zest

Toppings:

- √ 1–2 tablespoons crushed almonds
- √ Coconut flakes

Preparation Time: 10 minutes

Cooking Time: 0 minutes

Servings: 2

Difficulty: Easy

Directions:

In a bowl or container, all pudding ingredients must be mixed and chill overnight. To make sauce, puree raspberry sauce ingredients in a food processor. In a glass or mason jar, layer the chia seed pudding with the raspberry sauce. Top the parfait with crushed almonds and coconut shreds.

Nutrition:

Calories: 243

Fat: 8.8g

Fiber: 4.1g

Carbs: 19.5g

Protein: 4.4g

136. Broiled Pineapples with Vanilla Ice-cream

Ingredients:

- √ 8 ounces gluten-free vanilla ice-cream (Breyer's)
- √ 1 cup pineapple chunks
- √ 2 tbsp brown sugar or honey

Dairy-free/ Vegan

Preparation Time: 5 minutes

Cooking Time: 5-10 minutes

Servings: 2

Directions:

Difficulty: Easy

Preheat oven to broiler setting. Stir sugar or honey with pineapple.

Broil pineapple until slightly browned, approximately 10 minutes. Serve with gluten-free vanilla ice-cream.

Nutrition:

Calories: 151

Fat: 3.9g

Fiber: 4.9g

Carbs: 15.4g

Protein: 3.1g

137. Apple Pear Crisp

Ingredients:

- √ 3 medium pears
- √ 3 large apples

Other ingredients:

- √ 3/4 cup brown sugar

Dairy-free/ Vegetarian-friendly

Preparation Time: 15 minutes

Cooking Time: 40 minutes

Servings: 8

Difficulty: Easy

- √ teaspoon vanilla extract
- √ 1/2 cup rice flour
- √ 1/4 cup gluten-free oats
- √ 1/4 cup olive oil

Directions: Oven: 400°F

Peel and thinly slice pears and apples. In a bowl or container, combine other ingredients. Set aside. Spray a 2-quart casserole with cooking spray. Spread fruit in the bottom of a casserole. Top with sugar mixture. Let the crisp apple bake for about 40 minutes.

Nutrition:

Calories: 201

Fat: 9.8g

Fiber: 4.9g

Carbs: 16.6g

Protein: 3.1 g

138.   Peach and Raspberry Fruit Leather

Ingredients:

- √ 1 cup peaches
- √ 1 cup raspberries
- √ 1 – 2 teaspoons honey to taste

Dairy-free/ Vegan

Preparation Time: 15 minutes

Cooking Time: 3 hrs.

Servings: 8

Directions:

Difficulty: Easy

Oven: 200° F

Line a baking sheet with a Silpat. In a blender, add all ingredients and blend until smooth. Spread the mixture equally into a rectangular shape onto your Silpat. Bake for 2 – 3 hours until dry.

Nutrition:

Calories: 205

Fat: 5.9g

Fiber: 5.1g

Carbs: 17.4g

Protein: 4.3g

139.   Caramel Baked Apples

Ingredients:

- √ 4 medium apples, cored
- √ 4 dates
- √ 4 teaspoons salted pumpkin seeds, divided
- √ 4 teaspoons dairy-free butter, divided
- √ teaspoon ground cinnamon, divided

Dairy-free/ Vegan

Preparation Time: 10 minutes

Cooking Time: 40 minutes

Servings: 4

Difficulty: Medium

Directions: Oven: 375°F . Place the cored apples in an 8-by-8-inch baking dish.

Place 1 date in the center of each apple and top each with 1 teaspoon of pumpkin seeds, 1 teaspoon of butter, and ¼ teaspoon of cinnamon.

Carefully pour 1 cup of water around the apples in the bottom of the pan. Using aluminum foil, cover and bake for 20 minutes. Take the foil out and let it bake for 20 more minutes.

Nutrition:

Calories: 254

Fat: 15g

Fiber: 9.5g

Carbs: 29.5g

Protein: 3.1g

140.   Blackberry Cobbler

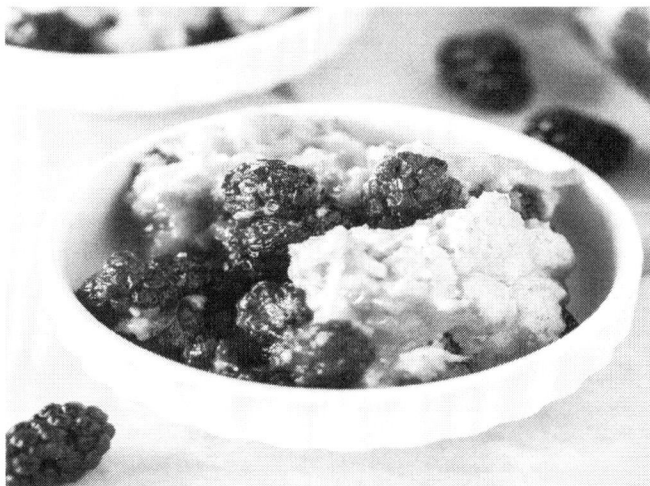

Ingredients:

- √ Shortening, for preparing the pan
- √ 250 grams white sugar
- √ 125 grams of rice flour
- √ 1½ teaspoons baking powder
- √ ½ teaspoon xanthan gum
- √ ½ teaspoon salt
- √ cup coconut milk
- √ 4 tablespoons coconut oil
- √ ½ teaspoon vinegar

Topping:

- √ 230 grams blackberries
- √ 2 tablespoons sugar

Dairy-free/ Vegan

Preparation Time: 150 minutes
Cooking Time: 60 minutes
Servings: 8
Difficulty: Easy

Directions: Oven: 350°F

Grease a 9-by-13-inch baking dish with shortening. In a bowl or container, combine all ingredients except the topping ingredients. The batter must be poured into the prepared baking dish. Arrange the blackberries on top and sprinkle the sugar on top.Bake for 50 minutes.

Nutrition:

Calories: 225

Fat: 9.5g

Fiber: 8.1g

Carbs: 16.4g

Protein: 3.1g

141.   Quinoa Fruit Salad

Ingredients:

- √ 1 cup quinoa
- √ 2 cups of water
- √ Salt
- √ Lime zest

Dairy-free/ Vegan

Preparation Time: 30 minutes
Cooking Time: 20 minutes
Servings: 4
Difficulty: Easy

- √ Lime jucie
- √ 2 cups green grapes
- √ cup strawberries
- √ 1 cup blueberries
- √ 4 mint leaves

Directions:

In a heated pan, combine the quinoa, water, and salt. Let it simmer for 20 minutes.

Stir in the remaining ingredients and let it chill for about 20 minutes. Top with mint leaves.

Nutrition:

Calories: 218

Fat: 4.1g

Fiber: 7.4g

Carbs: 8.4g

Protein: 3.5g

142. Winter Fruit Compote

Ingredients:

Dairy-free/ Vegan

- √ 3 pears
- √ 1 can pineapple chunks
- √ 1 cup dried apricots
- √ 1/2 cup dried cranberries
- √ 3 tablespoons orange juice
- √ 2 tablespoons brown sugar
- √ 3 tablespoons tapioca starch
- √ 1/2 teaspoon ground ginger
- √ 1/4 teaspoon cardamom
- √ 1/2 teaspoon nutmeg
- √ 2 cups dark sweet cherries

Preparation Time: 15 minutes

Cooking Time: 3-4 hrs.

Servings: 8

Difficulty: Easy

Garnish:

- √ 1/2 cup toasted flaked coconut

√   1⁄2 cup pecans

Directions:

In a slow cooker, combine all ingredients except the garnishes, and cook for 3-4 hrs on high. Garnish with nuts and coconut flakes when serving.

Nutrition:

Calories: 171

Fat: 10.5g

Fiber: 4.9g

Carbs: 15.7g

Protein: 1.4g

143.   Mango Blueberry Crisp

Ingredients:

Fruit filling:

√   1 cup of sugar
√   1 tablespoon cornstarch
√   11⁄2 teaspoons cinnamon
√   2 mangoes
√   4 cups blueberries
√   2 teaspoons vanilla

Crumble:

√   cup gluten-free oats
√   1⁄2 cup rice flour
√   1⁄2 cup brown sugar
√   Nutmeg
√   1⁄2 cup coconut oil

Dairy-free/ Vegetarian-friendly

Preparation Time: 30 minutes

Cooking Time: 45 minutes

Servings: 12

Difficulty: Medium

Directions: Oven: 350°F

In a bowl or container, all fruit filling must be combined. Pour into a greased 8" × 8" baking dish and set aside. Next to make topping, stir together all crumble ingredients until coarse.

Sprinkle the topping over fruit in the baking dish and let the crisp bake for 40–45 minutes.

Nutrition:

Calories: 224

Fat: 11.1g

Fiber: 4.2g

Carbs: 31.7g

Protein: 2.4g

144.   Cherry Dump Cake

Ingredients: *Dairy-free/ Vegetarian-friendly*

Dry: **Preparation Time:** 15 minutes

- √   1/2 cup rice flour   **Cooking Time:** 40 minutes
- √   1/2 cup tapioca starch   **Servings:** 9
- √   1/2 cup sugar   **Difficulty:** Easy
- √   teaspoon baking powder
- √   1/2 teaspoon baking soda
- √   1/2 teaspoon xanthan gum
- √   1/4 teaspoon salt

Other ingredients:

- √   2 cans cherry pie filling
- √   8 ounces chopped walnuts or pecans
- √   1/2 cup coconut oil

Directions: Oven: 350°F . Heavily grease a 9" × 13" cake pan with oil.

In a bowl or container, the dry ingredients must be combined. Set aside. Pour filling into the cake pan. Sprinkle dry mixture evenly over the filling. Top with chopped nuts and drizzle the oil overall. Bake for 40 minutes.

Nutrition:

Calories: 216

Fat: 15.1g

Fiber: 4.9g

Carbs: 31.7g

Protein: 2.7g

145. Strawberry Rhubarb Pie

Ingredients:

Filling:

- √ 21⁄2 cups rhubarb
- √ 21⁄2 cups strawberries
- √ 11⁄2 cups sugar
- √ 3 tablespoons cornstarch
- √ teaspoon lemon zest
- √ 1⁄2 teaspoon lemon juice
- √ 1⁄2 teaspoon cinnamon
- √ teaspoon vanilla extract
- √ 1⁄4 cup water

Other ingredients:

- √ unbaked Gluten-Free Pie
- √ tablespoons coconut oil

Dairy-free/ Vegetarian-friendly

Preparation Time: 40 minutes

Cooking Time: 40 minutes

Servings: 6

Difficulty: Easy

Directions: Oven: 350° F

In a heated saucepan, all filling ingredients must be comcbined and cook over medium heat, for 7 minutes until mixture thickens. Pour mixture into the pie crust that has been pressed into a 9" pie pan. Evenly place slices coconut oil chunks over pie filling. Let the pie bake for 25–30 minutes

Nutrition:

Calories: 211

Fat: 6.5g

Fiber: 4.1g

Carbs: 26.9g

Protein: 5.7g

146. Cherry Cobbler

Ingredients:

Filling:

- √ 14½-ounce cherries
- √ ⅔ cup of sugar
- √ 1 tablespoon tapioca
- √ teaspoon almond extract

Topping:

- √ cup almond flour
- √ ½ cup sugar
- √ 1 teaspoon baking powder
- √ ½ teaspoon xanthan gum
- √ ¼ teaspoon salt
- √ ¼ cup coconut oil
- √ 1 egg
- √ 1 teaspoon lemon zest
- √ ⅓ cup almond milk
- √ 1 teaspoon vanilla extract

Preparation Time: 15 minutes

Cooking Time: 40 minutes

Servings: 6

Difficulty: Easy

Directions: Oven: 375°F. An 8-inch square pan must be greased with nonstick spray.

Filling: In a bowl or container, stir together all the ingredients. Spread evenly in the prepared pan.

The topping: Combine all ingredients in a bowl. Drop by tablespoonfuls onto the filling; the topping will spread out as it bakes. Sprinkle the topping with a tablespoon of sugar. Bake until the topping is browned, 35 to 40 minutes.

Nutrition:

Calories: 210

Fat: 8.5g

Fiber: 6.1g

Carbs: 17.5g

Protein: 3.4g

147.   Poached Pears with Caramel Sauce

Ingredients:

PEARS

- √   4 cups of water
- √   1 cup granulated sugar
- √   4 pears, peeled
- √   lemon, cut into 4 round slices

CARAMEL SAUCE

- √   ¼ cup brown sugar
- √   ¼ cup coconut milk
- √   2 tablespoons dairy-free butter
- √   ¼ teaspoon salt
- √   teaspoon vanilla extract

Dairy-free/ Vegan

Preparation Time: 15 minutes

Cooking Time: 40 minutes
Servings: 4
Difficulty: Medium

Directions:

In a heated saucepan, and add the water and granulated sugar. Stir to dissolve the sugar.

When the sugar is dissolved, completely submerge the pears in the liquid. Tuck the lemon slices around the pears.Simmer for 20 minutes, until tender all the way through. To test, carefully pierce the largest part of a pear with a sharp paring knife.

SAUCE:

In a heated saucepan, cook all ingredients for 5 minutes. To serve, place each pear in a dessert bowl and spoon sauce over it.

Nutrition:

Calories: 237

Fat: 9.5g

Fiber: 7.9g

Carbs: 27.1g

Protein: 3.1 g

148.   Peach Galette

Ingredients:

- √ 1½ cups almond flour
- √ 2 tablespoons tapioca flour
- √ ¼ teaspoon of salt
- √ 1 egg, divided
- √ 3 tablespoons coconut oil
- √ 5 teaspoons cold water
- √ 8 peaches, thinly sliced
- √ teaspoon sugar

Dairy-free/ Vegetarian-friendly

Preparation Time: 15 minutes

Cooking Time: 15 minutes

Servings: 6

Difficulty: Easy

Directions: Oven: 400°F.

Combine dry ingredients in the food processor.

Transfer 1 tablespoon of the whisked egg to a small cup and set aside. Add the remaining egg and the coconut oil to the processor. Blend for a few seconds, just until integrated. Add cold water and blend just until the dough forms a ball. Flatten the dough into a 10-inch circle. Remove the top sheet of parchment paper.

Lay the slices of peaches in a circular pattern in the center of the tart. Fold the crust' edges over the peaches and pleat extra all the way around. Mix the reserved egg with the remaining 1 tablespoon cold water and brush the crust with it.

Sprinkle the sugar over the crust. Bake for 15 minutes.

Nutrition:

Calories: 243

Fat: 11.5g

Fiber: 6.9g

Carbs: 18.5g

Protein: 3.4g

Chapter 11. <u>FAST AND CHEAP SNACKS</u>

149.   Pao De Queijo

Ingredients:

Dairy-free/ Vegetarian-friendly

- √ 2 cups tapioca starch
- √ 1 Tbsp. sugar
- √ 1 tsp. salt
- √ 2 tsp. baking powder
- √ 2 eggs
- √ 5½ Tbsp. avocado oil
- √ ¾ cup of coconut milk
- √ 12 oz. ricotta cheese
- √ ½ cup dairy-free cheese

Preparation Time: 20 minutes

Cooking Time: 20 minutes

Servings: 12

Difficulty: Easy

Directions: Oven: 400°F

Mix all dry ingredients. Using a stand mixer combine eggs, butter, and milk. On low speed, blend in the dry ingredients. Add both types of cheese and mix for an additional 2 minutes or so. Let the dough rest for 20 minutes. Roll dough into balls and place on a cookie sheet. Let the balls bake for 20 minutes.

Nutrition:

Calories: 150

Fat: 10.5g

Fiber: 1.5g

Carbs: 10.2g

Protein: 1.8g

150.   Banana Fudge Pops

Ingredients:

Vegetarian-friendly

- √ 1 cup almond milk
- √ 2 ripe bananas
- √ 2 Tbsp. Cocoa powder
- √ ½ tsp. vanilla

Preparation Time: 20 minutes

Cooking Time: 15 minutes

Servings: 12

Difficulty: Easy

√   2 Tbsp. pecans or sunflower seeds

Directions:

All ingredients except for nuts must be placed in a blender and puree until smooth. Stir in nuts. Transfer to a popsicle maker and place it in the freezer. Chill at least 3 hours.

Nutrition:

Calories: 133

Fat: 2.7g

Fiber: 5.8g

Carbs: 14.4g

Protein: 1.2g

151.   Cinnamon and Sugar Donut Holes

Ingredients: *Dairy-free/ Vegetarian-friendly*

√   1 cup Gluten-free Pancake Mix   **Preparation Time:** 15 minutes
√   1 large egg   **Cooking Time:** 15-20 minutes
√   1 Tbsp. coconut oil oil   **Servings:** 10
√   ½ cup of water   **Difficulty:** Easy

For frying:

√   2 cups canola oil

Directions:

In a bowl or container, whisk all the ingredients together. Pour 2 cups oil into a skillet and heat on high. Drop dough into the pan by the tablespoon. Cook until all sides are golden brown.

Place cinnamon and sugar into a large plastic bag. Place the cooled donuts in the bag, seal, and shake until thoroughly coated.

Nutrition:

Calories: 215

Fat: 9.5g

Fiber: 4.4g

Carbs: 18.5g

Protein: 2.1 g

152. Baked Tater Tots

Ingredients:

Vegetarian-friendly

- √ 2 cups gluten-free potato chips
- √ 4 baked potatoes
- √ 1 egg
- √ 2 Tbsp. vegan butter
- √ tsp. salt
- √ ½ tsp. pepper
- √ ¼ cup grated onion

Preparation Time: 15 minutes

Cooking Time: 40 minutes

Servings: 15

Difficulty: Easy

Directions: Oven: 375°F

Line a baking sheet with parchment paper. Crush potato chips into a shallow dish. Grate into a bowl the peeled potatoes. Stir in remaining ingredients.

Make it into tater tots by taking a tablespoon of filling and push through a 1-inch ring mold. Roll in crushed chips. Place on a baking sheet and bake for 40 minutes.

Nutrition:

Calories: 201

Fat: 11g

Fiber: 3.1g

Carbs: 18.5g

Protein: 1.5 g

153. Cloud Bread

Ingredients:

Dairy-free/ Vegetarian-friendly

- √ 3 Tbsp. cream cheese
- √ 2 tsp. sugar
- √ 3 eggs, separated
- √ ¼ tsp. cream of tartar

Preparation Time: 15 minutes

Cooking Time: 25 minutes

Servings: 8

Difficulty: Easy

Directions: Oven: 300°F

In a bowl or container, mix the sugar and cream cheese until smooth. Add yolks one at a time and mix thoroughly.

In another bowl or container, beat egg whites and cream of tartar until they form stiff peaks. Carefully fold the egg yolk mixture into the egg whites. The mixture will be scooped into 8 rounds on the sheets. Let it bake for 30 minutes.

Nutrition:

Calories: 100

Fat: 3.1

Fiber: 1.5g

Carbs: 1.7g

Protein:2. 7g

154.   Tex Mex Tacos

Ingredients:

- √   2 slicesbacon
- √   ½ cup bell pepper
- √   ⅓ cup onion
- √   1 tablespoon jalapeño
- √   ½ tablespoon olive oil
- √   4 eggs
- √   Dash of salt

Other ingredients:

- √   4 corn tortillas
- √   avocado, sliced
- √   cilantro, minced
- √   fresh salsa

Dairy-free

Preparation Time: 10 minutes

Cooking Time: 10 minutes

Servings: 2

Difficulty: Easy

Directions:

In a skillet, sauté the bacon until it becomes crispy. Remove the bacon from the skillet.Now add in the remaining ingredients aside from the toppings. Add the bacon back into the skillet along with the eggs and seasonings. Warm each corn tortilla Fill the tortillas with the egg filling, then top each taco with other toppings.

Nutrition:

Calories: 215

Fat: 12.6g

Fiber: 3.1g

Carbs: 16.5g

Protein: 3.1 g

155.   Fruit Kabobs

Ingredients:

Dairy-free/ Vegan

- √   1/4 cup cantaloupe
- √   1/4 cup honeydew
- √   1/4 cup pineapple
- √   1/4 cup peach
- √   Small plastic straws

Preparation Time: 10 minutes

Cooking Time: 0 minutes

Servings: 6

Difficulty: Easy

Directions:

Cut each fruit into 1" cubes. Thread cubes onto the straw, alternating fruits.

Nutrition:

Calories: 110

Fat: 1.3f

Fiber: 5g

Carbs: 7g

Protein: 1.1g

156.   Black Bean Tortilla

Ingredients:

Dairy-free/ Vegetarian-friendly

Filling ingredients:

- √   1 teaspoon olive oil

Preparation Time: 15 minutes

Cooking Time: 10 minutes

- √ 1/4 cup onions, minced
- √ 1 teaspoon garlic, minced
- √ can black beans, rinsed and drained
- √ 4 ounces carrot purée
- √ 1 teaspoon cumin

Servings: 6
Difficulty: Easy

Other ingredients:

- √ 6 corn tortillas
- √ 1/2 avocado, mashed

Directions:

Heat olive oil in a skillet. Add all the filling ingredients. Heat tortillas in a dry skillet over medium heat. Top each tortilla with a thin layer of bean spread and then mashed avocado.

Nutrition:

Calories: 211

Fat: 10.6g

Fiber: 4.3g

Carbs: 21.7g

Protein: 5.4 g

157.   Cheesy Tomato Quesadilla

Ingredients:

Vegetarian-friendly

- √ 1/2 ripe avocado, mashed
- √ 2 corn tortillas
- √ 1 ripe tomato
- √ 1/4 cup non-dairy cheese
- √ 1/4 cup salsa

Preparation Time: 5 minutes
Cooking Time: 10 minutes
Servings: 1-2
Difficulty: Easy

Directions:

Add avocado mash on the tortilla. Dice tomato and layer on top of the avocado. Sprinkle cheese on top of this layer and top with the second tortilla. Place quesadilla in skillet. Heat until cheese begins to melt. Flip and cook to a golden brown. Top with salsa and serve.

Nutrition:

Calories: 155

Fat: 10.5g

Fiber: 4.5g

Carbs: 15.7g

Protein: 1.5g

158. Cornmeal Crusted Black Bean Bites

Ingredients: *Dairy-free/ Vegetarian-friendly*

- √ 1 can black beans, drained and rinsed   **Preparation Time:** 15 minutes
- √ egg or 1 tablespoon of ground flaxseeds mixed with 3 tablespoons warm water
- √ 1/4 cup cornmeal   **Cooking Time:** 15 minutes
- √ 1 teaspoon garlic pepper   **Servings:** 12
- √ 1/2 teaspoon salt   **Difficulty:** Easy
- √ 3–4 tablespoons olive oil, divided

Directions: Oven: 425°F

In a bowl or container, mash black beans and mix with egg or flaxseed gel. Scoop out mixture into 24 round balls. Combine cornmeal, garlic pepper, and salt in a bowl.

Dredge each beanball through the cornmeal, until they are thoroughly coated.

Spread 1 tablespoon olive oil on a cookie sheet or line with a sheet of parchment paper. Brush remaining olive oil gently over each ball. Bake black bean bites for 10–15 minutes.

Nutrition:

Calories: 154

Fat: 11.5g

Fiber: 4.1g

Carbs: 19.5g

Protein: 1.2g

159.   Parmesan Potato Wedges

Ingredients:

Dairy-free/ Vegetarian-friendly

- √ 4 potatoes, cut into wedges
- √ 2 tablespoons olive oil
- √ 1 tablespoon salt
- √ ¼ cup Parmesan cheese

Preparation Time: 10 minutes

Cooking Time: 30 minutes

Servings: 4

Difficulty: Easy

Directions: Oven: 450°F

Toss the potato wedges with the olive oil and salt on the sheet pan. Spread out the wedges in a single layer. Bake for 30 minutes. Sprinkle the Parmesan cheese over the wedges and bake for 5 more minutes.

Nutrition:

Calories: 161

Fat: 11.5g

Fiber: 3.1g

Carbs: 17.4g

Protein: 1.2g

160.   Cheesy Ham and Pickle Roll-ups

Ingredients:

Dairy-free

- √ 4 ounces cream cheese or non-dairy alternative
- √ 6 ounces sliced ham
- √ ½ cup pickle spears
- √ 3 scallions

Preparation Time: 15 minutes

Cooking Time: 0 minutes

Servings: 4

Difficulty: Easy

Directions:

A tablespoon of cream cheese must be spread on each slice of ham. Place a pickle and scallion at one end of each ham slice and roll it up into a tube shape. Cut each roll-up into 4 pieces.

Nutrition:

Calories: 161

Fat: 5g

Fiber: 3.5g

Carbs: 18.7g

Protein: 5.7g

161.　Italian Sausage Pizza

Ingredients:

Dairy-free

- √　1-pound Italian sausage, removed from casing
- √　1/4 cup onion
- √　1/2 cup green pepper
- √　1/2 teaspoon basil
- √　1/2 teaspoon oregano
- √　1/4 teaspoon salt
- √　1/2 cup grated Parmesan cheese or dairy-free substitute
- √　2 tomatoes

Preparation Time: 40 minute

Cooking Time: 40 minutes

Servings: 8

Difficulty: Medium

Dough Mix:

- √　cup gluten-free flour
- √　11/2 cups almond milk
- √　eggs

Other ingredients:

- √　cup shredded mozzarella cheese or dairy-free shredded cheese substitute

Directions: Oven: 350° F. Grease a 9" pie pan or large baking dish.

In a heated skillet, brown sausage, onion, and green pepper for 8–10 minutes.

Sprinkle drained sausage mixture, basil, oregano, garlic salt, Parmesan cheese, and tomatoes into pie pan. In a bowl or container, dough mix ingredients must be combined well. Pour batter over the pizza mixture. Sprinkle mozzarella cheese on top of the pie. Bake pie for 25–30 minutes.

Nutrition:

Calories: 265

Fat: 11.5g

Fiber: 5.5g

Carbs: 31.2g

Protein: 5.1g

162. Beef Tamale Pie

Ingredients:

Filling:

- √ 1-pound ground beef
- √ 1 cup canned corn
- √ 14 1/2-ounces diced tomatoes
- √ 2 1/4-ounce black olives
- √ 2 tablespoons gluten-free baking flour
- √ tablespoon chili powder
- √ teaspoons cumin
- √ 1/2 teaspoon salt

Crust:

- √ cup gluten-free baking flour
- √ 1/2 tsp baking soda
- √ 1/2 cup cornmeal
- √ 3/4 cup almond milk
- √ 1 egg

Dairy-free

Preparation Time: 15 minutes

Cooking Time: 25-30 minutes

Servings: 8

Difficulty: Easy

Directions: Oven: 400°F

Brown ground beef in a skillet until beef is cooked through. In a medium bowl, mix beef and remaining filling ingredients. Stir together well and pour the mixture into the pie pan.

In another medium bowl, whisk together the crust ingredients and pour over the ground beef mixture. Let the tamale pie bake for 25–30 minutes.

Nutrition:

Calories: 1218

Fat: 6.5g

Fiber: 3.1g

Carbs: 31.1g

Protein: 8.5g

163.　　Sesame Seed Wafers

Ingredients:

Dairy-free/ Vegetarian-friendly

- √　1 cup brown sugar
- √　1/4 cup coconut oil
- √　1 large egg
- √　1 teaspoon lemon juice
- √　1/2 teaspoon vanilla extract
- √　1/2 cup rice flour
- √　1/4 teaspoon salt
- √　1/8 teaspoon baking powder
- √　cup toasted sesame seeds

Preparation Time: 15 minutes

Cooking Time: 60 minutes

Servings: 10

Difficulty: Easy

Directions: Oven: 325°F

In a container or bowl, combine all ingredients and let it chill in the refrigerator for 30 minutes. Put dough by tablespoonfuls on the baking sheets and bake it for about 15 minutes.

Nutrition:

Calories: 112

Fat: 1.5g

Fiber: 1.9g

Carbs: 11.7g

Protein: 1.3g

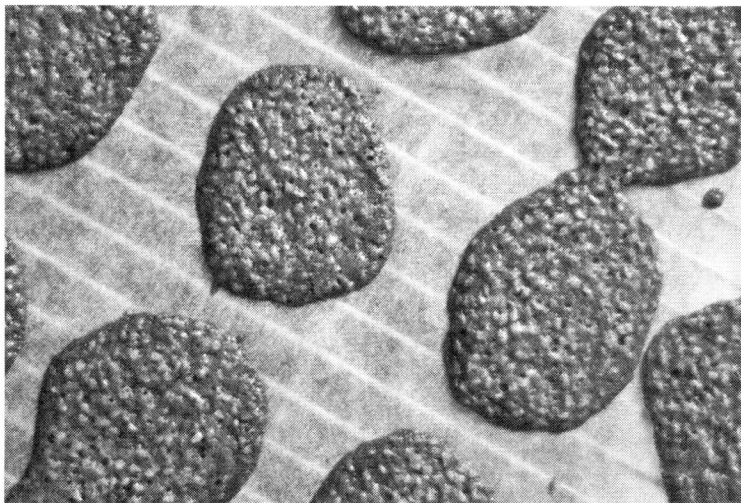

164.   Corn Dogs

Ingredients:

- √ 4 hot dogs' gluten-free
- √ 1/2 cup cornmeal
- √ 1/4 cup gluten-free flour
- √ 1 teaspoon sugar
- √ 1/2 teaspoon salt
- √ 1/4 teaspoon baking soda
- √ 1/2 cup almond milk
- √ 1/2 tablespoon vinegar
- √ egg
- √ 1 tablespoon oil
- √ 1 cup dairy-free cheese, optional

Dairy-free

Preparation Time: 15 minutes

Cooking Time: 12 minutes

Servings: 4

Difficulty: Easy

Directions: Oven: 425°F

Slice each hot dog into 6 even pieces; set aside. In a mixing bowl, whisk dry ingredients together, then add liquids and stir to combine. If desired, add cheese, then stir. Dividing evenly, spoon mixture into the pan and then add a piece of hot dog to each. Bake for 12 minutes.

Nutrition:

Calories: 150

Fat: 3.1g

Fiber: 4.1g

Carbs: 15.1g

Protein: 4.1g

165.   Fish Sticks

Ingredients:

- √ 1-pound cod fillets
- √ 2 eggs

DRY:

- √ 1/3 cup rice flour

Dairy-free

Preparation Time: 15 minutes

Cooking Time: 10-15 minutes

Servings: 4

Difficulty: Medium

√ 1/3 cup potato starch

√ ½ teaspoon salt

√ ¼ teaspoon pepper

OTHER INGREDIENT:

√ cup almond meal

Directions: Oven: 400°F

Cut the fish into strips about ½ to ¾ inches wide. In a bowl or container, the eggs must be beaten. In another bowl or container, combine dry ingredients. Put almond meal in the third container or bowl. Coat each fish with flour, dredge in the egg, and then finally on the almond meal. Let the fish sticks bake for 10 to 15 minutes.

Nutrition:

Calories: 211

Fat: 11.5g

Fiber: 3.1g

Carbs: 18.5g

Protein: 11g

166. Onion Rings

Ingredients:

√ 4 onions , cut into rings

Coating:

√ 3/4 cup gluten-free flour

√ 1/4 cup corn starch

√ 1/2 cup almond milk

√ 1/2 teaspoons salt

√ tablespoons vegetable oil

√ 1 egg white

√ tablespoons water

Dairy-free

Preparation Time: 15 minutes

Cooking Time: 15 minutes

Servings: 6

Difficulty: Medium

Directions:

Whisk all coating ingredients and set aside. Heat oil for frying. Dip onion rings in batter and fry until golden brown.

Nutrition:

Calories: 180

Fat: 8.5g

Fiber: 4.5g

Carbs: 16.7g

Protein: 1.4g

Chapter 12. <u>CAKES AND BREAD FOR KIDS</u>

167.   Mini Banana Loaves

Ingredients:

- √ 1/2 cup almond flour
- √ ¼ cup sorghum flour
- √ 3 Tbsp. rice flour
- √ ½ cup tapioca starch
- √ ¼ cup potato starch
- √ 2 Tbsp. coconut flour
- √ tsp. gelatin powder
- √ 1 tsp. baking power
- √ ½ tsp. salt
- √ ½ cup coconut oil
- √ 1 cup brown sugar
- √ eggs
- √ 1 tsp. vanilla extract
- √ 1 Tbsp. lemon juice
- √ ripe bananas, mashed
- √ ½ cup chopped walnuts (optional)

Preparation Time: 15 minutes

Cooking Time: 25 minutes

Servings: 4-6

Difficulty: Easy

Directions: Oven: 350° F

In a bowl or container, cream and combine all wet ingredients. Combine all dry ingredients. Add gradually.Pour the batter into the mini loaf pans and let the loaves bake for 25 minutes.

Nutrition:

Calories: 221

Fat: 4.6 g

Fiber: 4.1g

Carbs: 21.7g

Protein: 2.4 g

168.   Upside Down Pear Cake

Ingredients:

√   4 pears

Wet:

√   ½ cup almond milk
√   2 eggs
√   teaspoon vanilla extract
√   4 tablespoons honey, divided

Dry:

√   cup gluten-free flour
√   ½ cup almond meal
√   ½ cup of coconut sugar
√   teaspoons cinnamon
√   teaspoons baking powder
√   ½ teaspoon baking soda
√   ¼ teaspoon salt

Dairy-free/ Vegetarian-friendly

Preparation Time: 25 minutes

Cooking Time: 45 minutes

Servings: 12
Difficulty: Medium

Directions: Oven: 350° F

In a food processor, combine all wet ingredients. Process until smooth.

In a bowl or container, combine all dry ingredients. Combine the two mixture.

Slice the pears and arrange in a fan pattern on the bottom of a 9" cake pan. The batter must be poured over the pears. Let it bake for about 45 minutes. Serve and drizzle with honey.

Nutrition:

Calories: 231

Fat: 11.4g

Fiber: 5.3g

Carbs: 29.9g

Protein: 3.1g

169. Raspberry and Lemon Quick Bread

Ingredients:

Dry:

- √ ¾ cup of rice flour
- √ ½ cup sorghum flour
- √ ¼ cup potato starch
- √ tablespoon baking powder
- √ 1½ teaspoons xanthan gum
- √ tsp lemon zest
- √ ½ teaspoon baking soda
- √ ¼ teaspoon salt
- √ 1 cup granulated sugar

Wet:

- √ 2 eggs
- √ ½ cup coconut oil
- √ ½ cup sour cream
- √ 2 tablespoons lemon juice
- √ ½ teaspoon lemon extract
- √ 1½ cups raspberries

Dairy-free/ Vegetarian-friendly

Preparation Time: 15 minutes

Cooking Time: 60 minutes

Servings: 12

Difficulty: Easy

Directions: Oven: 350°F.

In a bowl or container, combine the sorghum flour, rice flour, potato starch, baking powder, xanthan gum, lemon zest, salt, and baking soda.

In a bowl or container, mix all wet ingredients. Put in the flour mixture. Carefully fold in the raspberries. Spoon the batter into the prepared pan. Let it bake for about 1 hour, covering with aluminum foil after 45 minutes of baking.

Nutrition:

Calories: 224

Fat: 9.5g

Fiber: 5g

Carbs: 33.7g

Protein: 4.3g

170. Orange and Pistachio Cake

Ingredients:

Cake:

- √ 2 cups gluten-free flour
- √ 1 tablespoon baking powder
- √ 2 tsp orange zest
- √ ½ teaspoon salt
- √ 2 large eggs
- √ ½ cup maple syrup
- √ ¾ cup orange juice
- √ ¼ cup avocado oil
- √ cup fresh cherries
- √ ¾ cup chopped pistachios

Glaze:

- √ cup confectioners' sugar
- √ 1 to 2 tablespoons orange juice
- √ 1 tsp orange zest

Dairy-free/ Vegetarian-friendly

Preparation Time: 15 minutes

Cooking Time: 55 minutes

Servings: 12

Difficulty: Easy

Directions: Oven: 375°F

In a bowl or container, combine all cake ingredients and carefully fold in the cherries and pistachios. Spoon into the prepared pan. Let it bake for about 55 minutes. In a container, whisk together all glaze ingredients. Drizzle over the bread.

Nutrition:

Calories: 241

Fat: 11.5g

Fiber: 4.1g

Carbs: 31.7g

Protein: 1.2g

171.   Strawberry Shortcake

Ingredients:

Cake:

- √ 2 tablespoons coconut flour
- √ 2 tablespoons almond flour
- √ 1 tablespoon granulated sugar
- √ ½ teaspoon baking powder
- √ Salt
- √ ¼ cup almond milk
- √ egg
- √ ¼ teaspoon strawberry extract

Garnish:

- √ cup sliced strawberries
- √   Whipped Cream

Vegetarian-friendly

Preparation Time: 10 minutes

Cooking Time: 2 minutes

Servings: 2

Difficulty: Easy

Directions:

In a bowl or container, combine all cake ingredients.Pour the dough into 1 or 2 coffee mugs and microwave on full power for 1 minute.

Let sit for 5 minutes. Serve the cake warm with slices of strawberries and whipped cream on top.

Nutrition:

Calories: 254

Fat: 11.2g

Fiber: 4.9g

Carbs: 33.2g

Protein: 3.1g

172.   Cinnamon Roll Cake

Ingredients:

CAKE:

- √ 3 cups gluten-free flour

Dairy-free/ Vegetarian-friendly

Preparation Time: 30 minutes

Cooking Time: 30 minutes

- √ ¼ teaspoon salt
- √ 1 cup granulated sugar
- √ 4 teaspoons baking powder
- √ 1½ cups almond milk
- √ 2 eggs
- √ 2 teaspoons vanilla extract
- √ ½ cup vegan butter

- √ cup coconut oil
- √ 1 cup brown sugar
- √ tablespoons gluten-free flour
- √ 1 tablespoon cinnamon

GLAZE

- √ 2 cups confectioners' sugar
- √ 5 tablespoons almond milk
- √ teaspoon vanilla extract

Servings: 16
Difficulty: Medium

Directions:

Oven: 350°F. Spray a 9" × 13" glass baking pan with gluten-free nonstick cooking spray.

In a bowl or container, add all cake ingredients. Pour into prepared baking pan. In another bowl or container, beat together the topping ingredients until smooth. Drop tablespoons of topping into the cake batter and use a knife to swirl it around. Let the cinnamon roll cake bake for 35–40 minutes. In a container or bowl, mix the glaze ingredients until smooth. Pour over warm cake and serve.

Nutrition:

Calories: 261

Fat: 10.9g

Fiber: 5g

Carbs: 34.1g

Protein: 1.7g

173.   Pineapple Upside Down Cake

Ingredients:

TOPPING

- √ ¼ cup coconut oil
- √ ⅔ cup brown sugar
- √ 20-ounce slice pineapple
- √ 9 maraschino cherries

CAKE

- √ ⅓ cup coconut oil
- √ cup of sugar
- √ 1 teaspoon vanilla extract
- √ 1 egg
- √ 1⅓ cups gluten-free flour
- √ 1½ teaspoons baking powder
- √ ½ teaspoon salt
- √ 1 cup almond milk

Dairy-free/ Vegetarian-friendly

Preparation Time: 35 minutes

Cooking Time: 50 minutes

Servings: 9

Difficulty: Hard

Directions:

Oven: 350°F. Spray a 9" × 9" pan with gluten-free nonstick cooking spray.

Pour oil into the bottom of the pan. Sprinkle brown sugar over it. Place pineapple slices on top of brown sugar and then place a cherry in the center of each pineapple slice. In a bowl or container, mix all cake ingredients and pour over the pineapple. Let it bake for about 50 minutes.

Nutrition:

Calories: 212

Fat: 11.4g

Fiber: 4.3g

Carbs: 31.4g

Protein: 1.2g

174.   Chocolate Zucchini Cake

Ingredients:

Dairy-free/ Vegetarian-friendly

- √ 5 tablespoons coconut oil, divided
- √ ½ cup brown sugar
- √ 4 eggs
- √ 1 tablespoon vanilla extract
- √ cup almond flour
- √ 1 tablespoon coconut flour
- √ ½ cup cocoa powder
- √ 1 teaspoon baking soda
- √ ½ teaspoon salt
- √ 1 zucchini, shredded

Preparation Time: 15 minutes
Cooking Time: 25 minutes
Servings: 8
Difficulty: Medium

Directions: Oven: 325° F . A 9-inch cake pan must be lined parchment paper.

In a bowl or container, add all wet ingredients and combine well. Stir in sifted dry ingredients and fold in the shredded zucchini. Pour the batter into the prepared pan. Let the zucchini bake, which will take for 25 minutes.

Nutrition:

Calories: 231

Fat: 9.5g

Fiber: 3.5g

Carbs: 31.1g

Protein: 2.1g

175.   Vanilla Berry Mug Cake

Ingredients:

Vegetarian-friendly

- √ Coconut oil (1 tbsp.)
- √ Cream cheese (2 tbsp.)
- √ Coconut flour (2 tbsp.)
- √ White Sugar (1 tbsp.)
- √ Vanilla extract (1 tsp.)

Preparation Time: 5 minutes
Cooking Time: 5 minutes
Servings: 1
Difficulty: Easy

- √ Baking powder (.25 tsp.)
- √ Egg (1)
- √ Raspberries (6)

Directions:

Combine all ingredients in a mug until smooth. Microwave it on medium for 5 minutes.

Nutrition:

Calories: 241

Fat: 11.1g

Fiber: 4.3gg

Carbs: 31.1g

Protein: 2.1g

176. Brownie Pecan Mug Cake

Ingredients:

Dairy-free/ Vegetarian-friendly

- √ Coconut oil (2 tbsp.)
- √ Almond flour (3 tbsp.)
- √ Salt (1 pinch)
- √ Coconut flour (1 tsp.)
- √ Sugar (1.5 tbsp.)
- √ Baking powder (.5 tsp.)
- √ Vanilla (.25 tsp.)
- √ Egg (1)
- √ cocoa powder (1 tbsp.)
- √ Chopped pecans (optional - 2 tbsp.)

Preparation Time: 5 minutes
Cooking Time: 5 minutes
Servings: 2
Difficulty: Easy

Directions:

Combine all ingredients in two mugs until smooth. Microwave it on medium for 5 minutes.

Nutrition:

Calories: 120

Fat: 9.5g

Fiber: 5g

Carbs: 31.4g

Protein: 2.3g

177.   Cinnamon Rolls

Ingredients:

- √ 21/2 cups almond flour
- √ 1/2 teaspoon baking soda
- √ 1/4 teaspoon sea salt
- √ 1/4 teaspoon cinnamon
- √ 1/4 cup shortening
- √ tablespoon honey
- √ 1/2 teaspoon vanilla extract
- √ eggs
- √ 2 teaspoons coconut flour
- √ 1/2 teaspoon vinegar

CINNAMON-WALNUT FILLING

- √ 1/2 cup walnut pieces
- √ 3 tablespoons honey
- √ tablespoon coconut oil
- √ 1/2 teaspoon vanilla extract
- √ 1 tablespoon cinnamon

Dairy-free

Preparation Time: 30 minutes

Cooking Time: 22 minutes

Servings: 6

Difficulty: Medium

Directions:

In a bowl or container, mix all dry ingredients.

In another bowl, whisk together all wet ingredients until smooth with no lumps remaining. Making use of a spoon, combine the wet and dry mixture. Put the dough in the chiller to cool for 30 minutes. Make filling by combining all ingredients in a food processor.

Once the dough is chilled, roll it out to about a 10 "× 12 "rectangle about 1/4 "thick. Drizzle top of the dough with the honey-cinnamon mixture. Then sprinkle top with walnut bits. Roll the dough into a tight log slowly then chill for an hour. Oven: 325°F

Cut the log into 1" rounds. Transfer the cinnamon roll biscuits to the baking sheet and bake about 18–22 minutes.

Nutrition:

Calories: 301

Fat: 11.9g

Fiber: 6.4g

Carbs: 31.2g

Protein:4.4 g

178.   Italian Cannoli

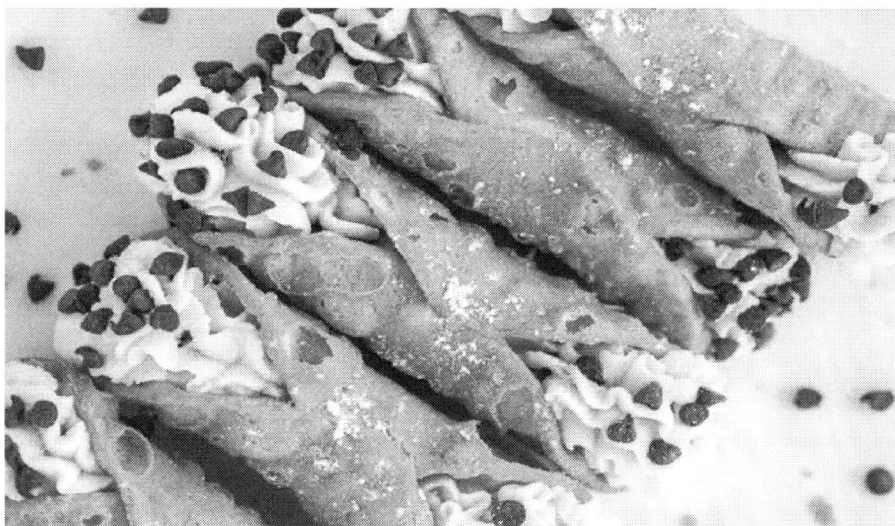

Ingredients:

SHELLS

- √   Shortening, for preparing the cannoli tubes
- √   313 grams gluten-free flour
- √   1½ tablespoons sugar
- √   teaspoon xanthan gum
- √   ¼ teaspoon salt
- √   tablespoons vegan butter
- √   egg yolks
- √   ⅔ cup white wine

Dairy-free/ Vegetarian-friendly

Preparation Time: 5 hrs.

Cooking Time: 25-30 minutes

Servings: 12

Difficulty: Hard

√ Oil, for frying

FOR THE FILLING

- √ 1,500 grams ricotta
- √ 2 teaspoons vanilla extract
- √ 150 grams of powdered sugar

Directions:

<u>Shells</u>: The baking sheet must be lined with parchment then set it aside. Then, on your working table, put a total of two parchment paper sheets, and dust them with flour. Grease 12 cannoli forms with shortening.

In a bowl or container, combine all shell ingredients. Shape it into a 12-inch log. Cut the log into 6 (2-inch) pieces. Roll each portion between the two sheets of parchment to ⅛ inch thick. Utilizing a 3-inch round biscuit or cookie cutter, cut out 1 round from each portion. Reroll the scraps and repeat. Carefully wrap each dough round around a cannoli form (or a tube made from aluminum foil). Your fingertip must then be dipped into the water to seal the seams. Do not wrap the dough too tightly, or they will be difficult to remove after frying.

Place all the cannoli shells on the prepared baking sheet and refrigerate for at least 4 hours.

Line a colander with paper towels, place it over a large bowl, and spoon the ricotta into the lined colander. Set over a bowl and refrigerate to drain for about 1 hour.

<u>To make the Filling</u>: In a container or bow, mix all filling ingredients. The filling will then be transferred to a piping bag and chill

<u>To finish the Cannoli</u>: Fry cannoli shells until golden brown. Fill the cannoli shells from both sides, making sure the middle gets filled. Dust the filled cannoli with powdered sugar.

Nutrition:

Calories: 177

Fat: 10.5g

Fiber: 4.1g

Carbs: 27.8g

Protein: 2.1g

179. Lemon Jelly Roll

Ingredients:

- √ Nonstick cooking spray
- √ 1⅓ cups gluten-free flour
- √ 1 teaspoon baking powder
- √ ½ teaspoon baking soda
- √ ¼ teaspoon salt
- √ ⅓ cup granulated sugar
- √ ¼ cup brown sugar
- √ 3 tablespoons coconut oil
- √ ¼ cup lemon juice
- √ 2 tablespoons lemon zest
- √ teaspoon vanilla extract
- √ eggs
- √ ½ cup coconut milk
- √ 1 cup confectioners' sugar
- √ tablespoons water
- √ 1 cup strawberry jam

Dairy-free/ Vegetarian-friendly

Preparation Time: 15 minutes
Cooking Time: 25 minutes
Servings: 8
Difficulty: Medium

Directions: Oven: 350°F. Two 8-inch cake pans must be coated with cooking spray.

In a bowl or container, all dry cake ingredients must be combined. In another bowl or container, all wet ingredients must be mixed. Slowly add the flour mixture and mix until combined.

Pour the batter into the pans.. Let the roll bake for about 20 to 25 minutes. In a bowl or container, mix the water and confectioners' sugar. The first cake layer must be spread with the jelly over the top, then place the remaining cake layer on top. Drizzle the sugar glaze over the cake and serve.

Nutrition:

Calories: 221

Fat: 5.7g

Fiber: 3.5g

Carbs: 31.7g

Protein: 3.7g

180.   Crunchy Breadsticks

Ingredients:

- √ 2¼ teaspoons instant rise yeast
- √ 1 tablespoon brown sugar
- √ ½ cup lukewarm water
- √ 1 large egg
- √ ½ cup sour cream
- √ tablespoon oil
- √ 1 teaspoon tarragon
- √ 1 teaspoon dill
- √ ½ teaspoon onion powder
- √ 1¾ cups Gluten-free flour
- √ ½ cup tapioca flour
- √ teaspoon salt

Dairy-free/ Vegetarian-friendly

Preparation Time: 35 minutes

Cooking Time: 20 minutes

Servings: 12

Difficulty: Medium

Directions:

The baking sheet must be lined with parchment then set it aside.

In a bowl or container, dissolve the sugar and yeast in the water. Stir with a fork until the yeast dissolves and let stand until the yeast foams.Whisk in the wet ingredients. Put in the dry ingredients an knead until it forms a dough. Cover with plastic wrap and set in a warm, draft-free place to rise for 45 minutes.

Preheat the oven to 350°F. Divide the dough into 24 balls. Roll each ball into 5-by-1-inch strips. Rise it for 25 minutes. Bake until golden brown, about 20 minutes.

Nutrition:

Calories: 101

Fat: 2.5g

Fiber: 1.2g

Carbs: 10.7g

Protein: 1.1g

181.   Lemon Pudding Cake

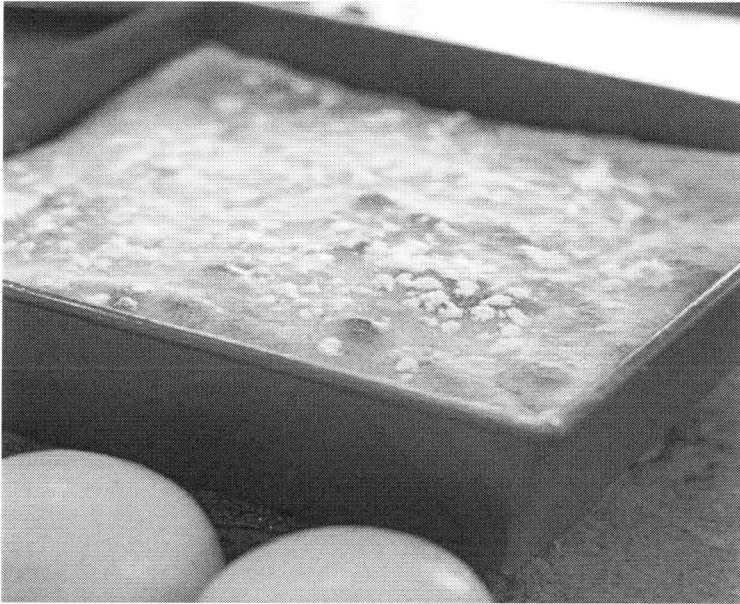

Ingredients:

Dairy-free/ Vegetarian-friendly

√   ¼ cup garbanzo bean flour

√   ¼ cup almond meal

√   ¼ cup arrowroot

√   ⅛ teaspoon salt

√   cup granulated sugar

√   1¼ cups coconut cream

√   4 tablespoons coconut oil

√   ⅓ cup lemon juice

√   Grated zest

√   teaspoon lemon extract

√   4 eggs

√   1 teaspoon cream of tartar

√   Dairy-free whipped cream, for topping

Preparation Time: 15 minutes

Cooking Time: 40 minutes

Servings: 6

Difficulty: Medium

Directions: Oven: 350° F

Place a roasting pan filled halfway with water in the oven. A 9-inch square baking pan must be coated with nonstick cooking spray. In a bowl or container, mix and combine all ingredients except eggwhites and cream of tartar.

In a bowl or container, egg whites and cream of tartar must be beaten until soft peaks form. Fold into the lemon mixture. Pour into the prepared pan. Carefully place the baking pan in the roasting pan in the oven. Bake for 40 minutes.

Nutrition:

Calories: 199

Fat: 5g

Fiber: 3.4g

Carbs: 29.7g

Protein: 1.2g

182. Sweet Potato Fries with Aioli Dip

Ingredients: *Dairy-free/ Vegetarian-friendly*

FRIES   **Preparation Time:** 15 minutes

- √ 3 sweet potatoes, cut into 1-by-4-inch fries   **Cooking Time:** 25-30 minutes
- √ 2½ tablespoons cornstarch   **Servings:** 4
- √ 4 tablespoons coconut oil   **Difficulty:** Medium
- √ ½ teaspoon salt
- √ ½ teaspoon pepper
- √ ½ teaspoon garlic powder

FOR THE AIOLI

- √ ½ cup Vegan Mayonnaise
- √ tablespoon lemon juice
- √ ½ teaspoon garlic powder

Directions: Oven: 400°F

The baking sheet must be lined with parchment then set it aside.

In a bowl or container, toss the sweet potatoes with the other ingredients. Gently toss the fries and spread them out in a single layer. Bake for 15 minutes. Flip the fries over and bake for 12 more minutes. In a bowl or container, mix the mayonnaise, lemon juice, and garlic powder.

Nutrition:

Calories: 171

Fat: 12.1g

Fiber: 3.1g

Carbs: 18.5g

Protein: 4.1g

183.   Deviled Eggs

Ingredients:

Dairy-free/ Vegetarian-friendly

- √ 6 eggs
- √ ¼ cup mayonnaise
- √ 2 teaspoons yellow mustard
- √ ½ teaspoon salt
- √ ⅛ teaspoon black pepper
- √ Paprika, for garnish
- √ Parsley and chives

Preparation Time: 25 minutes

Cooking Time: 10-15 minutes

Servings: 6

Difficulty: Easy

Directions:

Boil eggs for 5 minutes.Peel the eggs and cut each in half lengthwise. Set aside until completely cool. Remove the yolks and place them in a small bowl. Add the mayonnaise, mustard, salt, and pepper. Using a fork, mash the yolks to create a smooth mixture. Spoon or pipe the filling into the egg whites. Garnish with the paprika and fresh herbs.

Nutrition:

Calories: 151

Fat: 5.4g

Fiber: 2.5g

Carbs: 13.1g

Protein: 5.5 g

184.   Sugar Doughnuts

Ingredients:

Dairy-free/ Vegetarian-friendly

- √ 2 tablespoons Shortening

Preparation Time: 35 minutes

- √ 1⁄3 cup sugar
- √ 1 large egg
- √ 2 teaspoons vanilla extract
- √ 3⁄4 cup rice flour
- √ 1⁄2 cup arrowroot starch
- √ 1⁄2 teaspoon cinnamon
- √ 1⁄2 teaspoon baking powder
- √ 1⁄2 teaspoon baking soda
- √ 1⁄4 teaspoon sea salt
- √ 1⁄4 teaspoon xanthan gum
- √ 1⁄3 cup almond milk

Cooking Time: 8-10 minutes
Servings: 12
Difficulty: Medium

Coating:

- √ cup confectioners' sugar

Directions:

Oven: 350°F . A mini-doughnut pan must be sprayed with nonstick cooking spray.

In a bowl or container, cream together the sugar and shortening. Stir in the egg and vanilla and set aside. Add in other dry and wet ingredients.

Squeeze the batter into the doughnut pans. Bake 8–10 minutes. Once the doughnuts are cool, put confectioners' sugar in a large zip-top plastic bag. Add the doughnuts, seal the bag, and shake to coat all the doughnuts.

Nutrition:

Calories: 187

Fat: 11.5g

Fiber: 3.5g

Carbs: 31.1g

Protein: 1.5g

Chapter 13. <u>CAKES FOR EVENTS</u>

185.   Valentine Chocolate and Berries Cake

Ingredients:

Dairy-free/ Vegetarian-friendly

√ 2 cups pecans

√ 1 cup brown sugar

√ 4 eggs

√ ½ cup canola oil

√ 5 tablespoons cocoa powder

√ teaspoon vanilla extract

√ ⅛ teaspoon salt

Preparation Time: 20 minutes

Cooking Time: 45 minutes

Servings: 10

Difficulty: Medium

Garnish:

√ Powdered sugar

√ raspberries, strawberries and mint sprigs

Directions: Oven: 350° F. Grease a 9-inch nonstick springform pan

Grind the pecans to the consistency of pecan meal using a food processor. All the remaining ingredients must be added (except the garnishes) and blend for 30 to 40 seconds. Spread the batter in the pan. Let it bake for about 45 minutes. Slice and serve with a dusting of powdered sugar plus garnishes of fresh fruit and mint sprigs.

Nutrition:

Calories: 276

Fat: 12.5g

Fiber: 4.3g

Carbs: 31.1g

Protein: 2.1g

186.   Mexican Wedding Cookie Cake

Ingredients:

Dairy-free/ Vegetarian-friendly

√ ⅓ cup coconut oil

Preparation Time: 15 minutes

- √ ½ cup of sugar
- √ 1 tablespoon vanilla extract
- √ 2 teaspoons lemon zest
- √ 1½ cups Gluten-Free Flour
- √ ¼ cup cornstarch
- √ ¼ cup almond meal
- √ ¼ teaspoon xanthan gum
- √ ¼ teaspoon salt
- √ ⅛ teaspoon baking soda
- √ 2 tablespoons water

Cooking Time: 15 minutes

Servings: 12

Difficulty: Medium

Garnish:

- √ ½ cup powdered sugar

Directions: Oven: 375°F

Combine the sugar, coconut oil, vanilla, and lemon zest in a food processor. Process for 1 minute. Add the dry ingredients. Mix well. Add water and chill for two hrs.

Preheat the oven to 375°F. Line a 9x13-inch baking sheet with parchment paper. Put batter into the pan and let the cookie cake bake for 12 minutes. Dust powdered sugar before serving.

Nutrition:

Calories: 281

Fat: 11.5g

Fiber: 4.1g

Carbs: 32.3g

Protein: 3.1g

187.   Big Batch Yellow Sheet Cake for Birthdays

Ingredients:

Dairy-free/ Vegetarian-friendly

For greasing:

- √ ¼ teaspoon coconut oil

Preparation Time: 15 minutes

Cooking Time: 35 minutes

Substitute Buttermilk:

- √ 1 tablespoon vinegar
- √ 1¼ cups plus 3 tablespoons coconut milk

Dry:

- √ 345 grams gluten-free flour
- √ 1½ teaspoons baking powder
- √ 1½ teaspoons xanthan gum
- √ teaspoon salt
- √ ½ teaspoon baking soda
- √ 1½ cups granulated sugar

Wet:

- √ 3 large eggs
- √ ¾ cup sunflower oil
- √ tablespoon vanilla extract

Servings: 18

Difficulty: Medium

Directions: Oven: 350°F . Grease a 9-by-13-inch metal cake pan with oil.

In a measuring cup, put the vinegar first, then add enough coconut milk. Set aside

Place the dry ingredients in the bowl of a stand mixer. Mix then add the wet ingredients to the mixer. Pour the batter into the pan. Bake the yellow cake for 35 minutes.

Nutrition:

Calories: 287

Fat: 11.9g

Fiber: 4.1g

Carbs: 33.4g

Protein: 2.9g

188. **Afternoon Tea Party Cakes**

Ingredients:

Dry:

- √ 1 cup almond meal

Dairy-free/ Vegetarian-friendly

Preparation Time: 10 minutes

Cooking Time: 15 minutes

- √ ½ cup potato starch
- √ ¼ cup coconut flour
- √ teaspoon xanthan gum
- √ teaspoon baking powder
- √ ½ teaspoon baking soda
- √ ½ teaspoon salt

Wet:

- √ 2 eggs
- √ ¾ cup non-dairy yogurt
- √ ¾ cup honey
- √ teaspoon vanilla extract

Servings: 16
Difficulty: Medium

Directions: Oven: 350°F . A 24-cup mini muffin pan must be coated with nonstick cooking spray.

In a container or bowl, sift together all dry ingredients.

In another bowl or container, whisk together wet ingredients.Stir into the flour mixture just until combined. Fill the 24 mini muffin cups with the batter. Bake for 13 to 15 minutes.

Nutrition:

Calories: 243

Fat: 15g

Fiber: 4.1g

Carbs: 31.1g

Protein: 2.1g

189.   Simple Vanilla Birthday Cake

Ingredients:

Cake:

- √ 3¼ cups gluten-free flour
- √ ½ cup almond meal
- √ 1 tablespoon baking powder
- √ teaspoon baking soda

Dairy-free/ Vegetarian-friendly

Preparation Time: 25 minutes

Cooking Time: 25 minutes

Servings: 12

Difficulty: Medium

- √ 1 teaspoon xanthan gum
- √ 1 teaspoon salt
- √ ½ cup vegan butter
- √ cups granulated sugar
- √ 5 large eggs
- √ cup plain dairy-free yogurt
- √ teaspoons vinegar
- √ teaspoons vanilla extract

For the frosting:

- √ cup vegan butter
- √ ¼ to ½ cup dairy-free milk
- √ 1 tablespoon vanilla extract
- √ 5 cups confectioners' sugar

Directions: Oven: 350°F. Coat three 9-inch round cake pans with nonstick cooking spray.

In a medium bowl, combine all dry ingredients for the cake. In a bowl or container, cream the butter and sugar together until fluffy,then add remaining wet ingredients. Blend in the flour mixture. Pour into the pans. Bake for 20 to 25 minutes.

For the frosting, combine all ingredients together until smooth. Spread the frosting between the layers and frost the top and all sides of the cake.

Nutrition:

Calories: 291

Fat: 9.5g

Fiber: 4.1g

Carbs: 29.7g

Protein: 2.1 g

190.   Valentine's Day Cake with Cream Cheese Frosting

Ingredients:

Cake:

- √ 2 cups gluten-free flour

Vegetarian-friendly

Preparation Time: 25 minutes

Cooking Time: 25 minutes

- √ ½ cup almond meal
- √ ¼ cup cocoa powder
- √ tablespoon baking powder
- √ 1 teaspoon baking soda
- √ 1 teaspoon xanthan gum
- √ teaspoon salt
- √ ½ cup of coconut oil
- √ cups light brown sugar
- √ 5 eggs
- √ 1 cup sour cream
- √ 1 ounce red food coloring
- √ teaspoons vinegar
- √ 2 teaspoons vanilla extract

Servings: 12
Difficulty: Medium

For the frosting:

- √ cup of coconut oil
- √ 8 ounces cream cheese
- √ 1 tablespoon vanilla extract
- √ 5 cups confectioners' sugar

Directions:

Oven: 350°F . Three 9-inch round cake pans must be sprayed with nonstick cooking spray.

In a medium bowl, combine all dry ingredients for the cake. In a bowl or container, cream the butter and sugar together until fluffy,then add remaining wet ingredients. Blend in the flour mixture. Pour into the pans. Bake for 20 to 25 minutes

For the frosting, combine all ingredients together until smooth. Spread the frosting between the layers and frost the top and all sides of the cake.

Nutrition:

Calories: 299

Fat: 11.5g

Fiber: 4.1g

Carbs:31.4g

Protein: 1.1g

191.   Wedding White Cake

Ingredients:

CAKE

- √ ⅔ cup of coconut oil
- √ 1⅔ cups granulated sugar
- √ 1 teaspoon almond extract
- √ 2¼ cups gluten-free flour
- √ 3½ teaspoons baking powder
- √ ½ teaspoon salt
- √ 1½ cups almond milk
- √ 5 egg whites

BUTTERCREAM

- √ cup vegan butter
- √ 1½ teaspoons vanilla extract
- √ ¼ teaspoon almond extract
- √ 4 cups confectioners' sugar

Dairy-free/ Vegetarian-friendly

Preparation Time: 15 minutes

Cooking Time: 25-30 minutes

Servings: 16

Difficulty: Medium

Directions: Oven: 350°F. Two 8" cake pans and spray with nonstick cooking spray.

In a container or bowl, beat together the sugar and coconut oil on medium speed until smooth. Add remaining ingredients except the egg whites. Beat in the egg whites and combine on high for about 2 minutes. Divide the batter evenly between prepared cake pans. Bake on the middle rack for 28 minutes.

In a bowl or container, beat the vegan butter at medium speed until smooth. Add vanilla and almond extracts. Mix until fully combined. Put in confectioners' sugar a cup at a time and mix until combined. Cool cakes in the pans for about 10–15 minutes. Frost the cake.

Nutrition:

Calories: 287

Fat: 10.4g

Fiber: 4.3g

Carbs: 31.4g

Protein: 1.8g

192.   Southern Hummingbird Wedding Cake

Ingredients:

Dairy-free/ Vegetarian-friendly

- √ ⅓ cup almond milk
- √ 1 teaspoon vinegar
- √ 1 cup vegan butter
- √ 2 cups granulated sugar
- √ 4 eggs
- √ tablespoon vanilla extract
- √ cups gluten-free flour
- √ ½ teaspoon baking powder
- √ 1 teaspoon baking soda
- √ 1 teaspoon cinnamon
- √ 1 teaspoon salt
- √ ripe bananas mashed
- √ 8-ounce crushed pineapple
- √ 1 cup pecans

Preparation Time: 15 minutes
Cooking Time: 30 minutes
Servings: 16
Difficulty: Hard

FROSTING

- √ cup butter
- √ (8-ounce) packages dairy-free cream cheese
- √ tablespoons lemon juice
- √ tablespoon vanilla extract
- √ cups confectioners' sugar

Topping:

- √ ½ cup chopped pecans

Directions: Oven: 350°F. Spray two 9" round cake pan with gluten-free nonstick cooking spray.

In a bowl or container, add vinegar and milk and allow to sit for 2–3 minutes to make buttermilk.

In a large bowl, cream together buttery spread and sugar until smooth. Add the eggs in gradually and vanilla extract and mix until fully combined. Put in the remaining ingredients and mix well. The batter must be divided into the two cake pans. Bake for 30–35 minutes. Make frosting by combining all ingredients Allow cake to completely cool before frosting. Frost cake and sprinkle the top with pecans.

Nutrition:

Calories: 290

Fat: 10.1g

Fiber: 4.1g

Carbs: 31.7g

Protein: 1.2g

193.   Christmas Frosted Coconut Cake

Ingredients:

Dairy-free/ Vegetarian-friendly

CAKE

Preparation Time: 15 minutes

- √   ⅔ cup of coconut oil
- √   1⅔ cups granulated sugar
- √   1 teaspoon almond extract
- √   2¼ cups gluten-free flour
- √   3½ teaspoons baking powder
- √   ½ teaspoon salt
- √   1½ cups coconut milk beverage
- √   2 cups coconut flakes
- √   5 egg whites

Cooking Time: 30 minutes
Servings: 12
Difficulty: Hard

FROSTING

- √   cup vegan butter
- √   1½ teaspoons vanilla extract
- √   ¼ teaspoon almond extract
- √   4 cups confectioners' sugar
- √   1 cup coconut flakes

Directions: Oven: 350°F. Two 8" cake pans must be sprayed with nonstick cooking spray.

In a bowl or container, beat together all ingrediens except the egg whites. Beat in the egg whites and mix it on high for about 2 minutes. Divide batter evenly between prepared cake pans. Bake on the middle rack for 28 minutes.

In a bowl or container, combine all frosting ingredients. Cool cakes and frost all sides of and top of the cake.

Nutrition:

Calories: 281

Fat: 10.5g

Fiber: 4.3g

Carbs: 33.1g

Protein: 2.1 g

---

194. Christmas Poke Cake

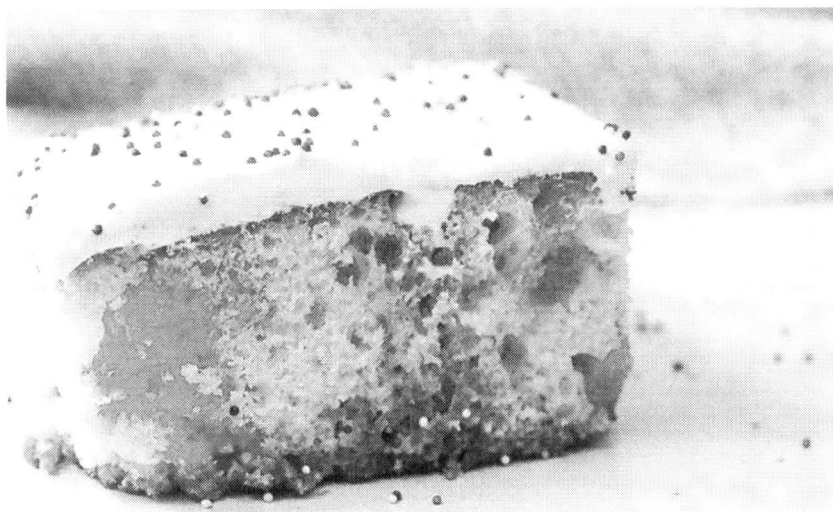

Ingredients:

- √   1 cup rice flour
- √   1 cup arrowroot starch
- √   1 cup of sugar
- √   2 teaspoon baking powder
- √   teaspoon baking soda
- √   1 teaspoon xanthan gum
- √   1/2 teaspoon salt
- √   1/2 cup canola oil
- √   11/2 cups almond milk
- √   4 large eggs

Dairy-free/ Vegetarian-friendly

Preparation Time: 30 minutes

Cooking Time: 30 minutes

Servings: 10-12

Difficulty: Medium

- √ tablespoon vanilla extract
- √ 3-ounce package strawberry or cherry gelatin
- √ 1 cup boiling water, divided
- √ 1⁄2 cup cold water, halved
- √ 1⁄2 (3-ounce) package lime gelatin
- √ 8-ounce whipped topping

Directions: Oven: 350°F . A 9" × 13" baking dish must be lined with parchment paper.

In a bowl or container, the dry ingredients must be mixed. In another bowl, whisk wet ingredients together thoroughly and then add to the dry ingredients. Pour cake mix into baking dish. Bake for 25–30 minutes. Once the cake has cooled, poke holes all around the top using a fork for tiny holes or the handle of a wooden spoon for larger holes.

Next, prepare gelatin mixtures. In a small bowl, mix the strawberry or cherry gelatin with 1⁄2 cup boiling water and 1⁄4 cup cold water. Pour mixture over the cake. In a bowl or container, continue by mixing the lime gelatin with 1⁄2 cup boiling water and 1⁄4 cup cold water and pour sporadically over the cake. Chill for at least 4 hours.

Frost cake with whipped topping.

Nutrition:

Calories: 213

Fat: 3.5g

Fiber: 1.5g

Carbs: 29.6g

Protein: 2.1g

195.   Thanksgiving Pumpkin Cheesecake

Ingredients:

Crust:

- √ 3⁄4 cup almond meal
- √ 1⁄2 cup ground pecans
- √ 2 tablespoons sugar

Dairy-free/ Vegetarian-friendly

Preparation Time: 30 minutes

Cooking Time: 55 minutes

Servings: 9

Difficulty: Medium

- √ 2 tablespoons brown sugar
- √ 1/4 cup coconut oil

Filling:

- √ 3/4 cup sugar
- √ 3/4 cup pumpkin purée
- √ 3 egg yolks
- √ 11/2 teaspoons cinnamon
- √ 1/2 teaspoon nutmeg
- √ 1/2 teaspoon ginger
- √ 1/4 teaspoon salt
- √ 3 (8-ounce) packages cream cheese
- √ 3/8 cup sugar
- √ egg
- √ 1 egg yolk
- √ tablespoons whipping cream
- √ 1 tablespoon cornstarch
- √ 1 teaspoon vanilla extract

Topping:

- √ 1/2 cup pecans
- √ 15-ounce dulce de leche

Directions: Oven: 350°F

Combine the crust ingredients and mix well. Firmly press into one 9" springform pan. Combine filling ingredients in another bowl. Mix well and set aside. Pour batter into prepared pan.

Bake for 50–55 minutes. Cover and refrigerate until ready to serve. Decorate cake top with whole pecans and dulce de leche.

Nutrition:

Calories: 298

Fat: 11.1g

Fiber: 4.1g

Carbs: 31.7g

Protein: 1.5g

---

196. Fourth of July Angel Food Cake

Ingredients:

Dairy-free/ Vegetarian-friendly

Cake:

Preparation Time: 30 minutes

- √ 1½ cups sugar, divided
- √ ¾ cup rice flour
- √ ½ cup potato starch
- √ ¼ cup tapioca flour
- √ 2 teaspoons xanthan gum
- √ 12 egg whites
- √ 1½ teaspoons vanilla extract
- √ ¼ teaspoon almond extract
- √ ½ teaspoon salt
- √ teaspoon cream of tartar

Cooking Time: 45 minutes

Servings: 12

Difficulty: Hard

For the coconut whipped cream and strawberries

- √ can coconut cream, chilled for 24 hours
- √ ½ cup confectioners' sugar
- √ ½ teaspoon vanilla extract
- √ 4 cups sliced strawberries

Directions: Oven: 325 °F

Do not grease the angel food cake pan. Sift ¾ cup of the sugar, the rice flour, potato starch, tapioca flour, and xanthan gum into a medium bowl.

In a bowl or container, beat the egg whites, vanilla, almond extract, and salt together until foamy. Blend in the cream of tartar and beat until soft peaks form. Continue beating while gradually add the remaining sugar, ¼ cup at a time, until incorporated. Beat it continuously until glossy, stiff peaks form. Sift one-third of the flour mixture over the egg white mixture. Carefully fold it in with a spatula until incorporated Pour the batter into the pan. Bake for 35 to 45 minutes. Turn the pan upside down on a wire rack.Let cool completely for 2 hours.

For the coconut whipped cream, beat all ingredients until fluffy.

Slice and serve the angel food cake with a dollop of whipped cream topped with the strawberries.

Nutrition:

Calories: 298

Fat: 10.4g

Fiber: 4.1g

Carbs: 31.4g

Protein: 1.5 g

197.   Independence Day Berry Layer Cake

Ingredients: *Dairy-free/ Vegan*

VANILLA CASHEW CREAM   **Preparation Time:** 30 minutes

- √   2 cups raw whole cashews, soaked in water overnight, drained and rinsed
- √   ½ cup almond milk   **Cooking Time:** 35 minutes
- √   ¼ cup maple syrup   **Servings: 12**
- √   1 teaspoon vanilla extract   **Difficulty:** Medium

COCONUT CREAM

- √   cup coconut cream
- √   1 tablespoon maple syrup
- √   ½ teaspoon vanilla extract

CAKE

- √   ¾ cup coconut milk
- √   teaspoon vinegar
- √   1½ cups = rice flour
- √   4 flax eggs (4 tablespoons ground flaxseed and 8 tablespoons water)
- √   1½ cups almond flour
- √   ¾ cup of coconut sugar
- √   tablespoons tapioca flour
- √   1½ teaspoons baking powder

- √ teaspoon baking soda
- √ ½ teaspoon of salt
- √ ¾ cup applesauce
- √ ⅓ cup maple syrup
- √ teaspoon vanilla extract
- √ tablespoons coconut oil

GARNISH

- √ 3 cups berries

Directions:

In a high-speed blender, blend all cashew cream ingredients until smooth. Transfer to a medium bowl.

To make the coconut whipped cream, use a hand mixer to beat the ingredients until fluffy. Combine the two mixture. This is the vegan mascarpone.

Oven: 325°F . Two 8-inch round springform cake pans must be coated with cooking spray.

In a bowl or container, prepare the flax eggs by mixing the ground flaxseed and water. Set aside for at least 10 minutes. In a bowl or container, you must combine the coconut milk and vinegar. Whisk and set aside. In a bowl or container, combine both dry and ingredients. Add in vinegared milk and flax eggs. The batter must be distributed to the cake pans; let the berry cake bake for 30-35 minutes.

Spread half of the vegan mascarpone on top of one cake, and place the second cake on top. Spread the remaining mascarpone on top. Decorate with the fresh berries.

Nutrition:

Calories: 291

Fat: 11.5g

Fiber: 4.1g

Carbs: 33.1g

Protein: 1.5 g

198.   New Year's Eve Moist Chocolate Cake

Ingredients: *Dairy-free*

CAKE   **Preparation Time:** 25 minutes

- √ 4 flax eggs (4 tablespoons ground flaxseed and 8 tablespoons water)

- √ 1 cup coconut milk
- √ 1 teaspoon vinegar
- √ 1½ cups rice flour
- √ cup almond flour
- √ ¾ cup of coconut sugar
- √ ½ cup cocoa powder
- √ 1½ teaspoons baking powder
- √ teaspoon baking soda
- √ ½ teaspoon of salt
- √ ½ cup pumpkin purée
- √ ⅓ cup maple syrup
- √ 1 teaspoon vanilla extract
- √ ¼ cup coconut oil

FROSTING

- √ can cococnut cream
- √ 1 teaspoon vanilla extract
- √ 1 cup of coconut sugar
- √ 1½ tablespoons arrowroot starch
- √ 1¼ cups shredded coconut
- √ cup chopped pecans

Cooking Time: 35 minutes
Servings: 12
Difficulty: Hard

Directions:

Oven: 350°F. Two 8-inch round springform cake pans must be coated with cooking spray.

In a bowl or container, make the flax eggs by mixing the water and ground flaxseed. Set aside for at least 10 minutes. In a medium bowl, combine the coconut milk and vinegar. Whisk and set aside.

In a bowl or container, combine all dry and wet ingredients. Add in vinegar-milk and flax eggs. The batter must be distributed to the prepared cake pans. Bake for 30 to 35 minutes.

In a medium saucepan over medium heat, mix the coconut milk and the vanilla, and bring to a boil. Whisk in the coconut sugar, and continue to cook for 1 to 2 more minutes. Add the arrowroot starch, and whisk well. stir in the chopped pecans and shredded coconut. Spread half of the frosting on top of one cake. Frost the remaining parts of the cake.

Nutrition:

Calories: 291

Fat: 9.8g

Fiber: 4.1g

Carbs: 31.1g

Protein: 1.8g

199.   Christmas Gingerbread Cake

Ingredients:

Dairy-free/ Vegan

- √ 1 cup almond flour
- √ 1 cup of rice flour
- √ 1 1/2 teaspoons baking soda
- √ 1 1/2 teaspoons ground ginger
- √ teaspoon xanthan gum
- √ 1/2 teaspoon salt
- √ 1/4 teaspoon cinnamon
- √ 1/2 cup coconut milk
- √ 1/2 teaspoon vinegar
- √ 3 tablespoons water
- √ tablespoon ground flaxseed meal
- √ 1 cup molasses
- √ 1/3 cup shortening
- √ 1/2 cup raisins
- √ tablespoons granulated sugar

Preparation Time: 20 minutes

Cooking Time: 40 minutes

Servings: 8

Difficulty: Easy

Directions: Oven: 325°F

Lightly grease a Bundt pan with canola oil.

In a medium mixing bowl, whisk all ingredients until smooth, Let the gingerbread cake bake, which can take for 55 minutes.

Nutrition:

Calories: 255

Fat: 11.5g

Fiber: 2.9g

Carbs: 29.9g

Protein: 3.1g

200. Halloween Death by Chocolate Cake

Ingredients:

CAKE

- √ Shortening, for preparing the pans
- √ 157 grams gluten-free flour
- √ 75 grams cocoa powder
- √ 62 grams arrowroot
- √ 2 teaspoons ground espresso
- √ 2 teaspoons baking soda
- √ teaspoon baking powder
- √ 1 teaspoon xanthan gum
- √ 1 teaspoon salt
- √ 350 grams sugar
- √ 1 cup oil
- √ large eggs
- √ cup almond milk
- √ 60 grams sour cream
- √ 1 shot brewed espresso
- √ tablespoons vanilla extract
- √ 1 teaspoon vinegar

CHOCOLATE FROSTING

- √ 136 grams shortening
- √ 720 grams of powdered sugar
- √ 75 grams cocoa powder
- √ 2 teaspoons vanilla extract
- √ 6 tablespoons coconut milk

Dairy-free/ Vegetarian-friendly

Preparation Time: 35 minutes

Cooking Time: 30 minutes

Servings: 8

Difficulty: Hard

Directions: Oven: 350° F. Grease two 9-inch springform pans with shortening.

In a bowl or container, all dry cake ingredients must be combined.

In another bowl or container, all wet ingredients must be mixe. Slowly add the flour mixture and mix until combined. Pour the batter into the pans. Let it bake for about 25 to 28 minutes.

Frosting: In a bowl or container, beat and cream all frosting ingredients.

Frost the cake layers and serve.

Nutrition:

Calories: 298

Fat: 11.4g

Fiber: 4.1g

Carbs: 31.1g

Protein: 1.5g

Conclusion

Gluten refers to the protein present in most grains, especially in barley, wheat, rye, and triticale. The gluten present in foods helps keep the food together and helps the food maintain its shape. Gluten can be found in a large number of food types. As discussed in the first part of this book, we now know that gluten is not good for people who have leaky guts or what we call celiac disease. People who are not able to tolerate gluten experience a variety of symptoms, which include constipation, passing gas, tingling, and so on. Due to the inconvenient symptoms gluten brings to a person, and how it destroys the digestive system, there's a need for a person to adapt to a gluten-free diet. A balanced gluten-free diet will also bring back the hormonal balance and condition your mind and body to "want" to lose weight. Your appetite will be tempered, and your cravings reduced.

That is where this book comes in. In these pages, you were given 200 great gluten-free snack and dessert recipes to aid in you getting started on your gluten-free diet. Not only that, but you were also provided with information that will aid you in gaining insight on how to have a full life free from gluten. To get your gluten-free diet into gear, you need to have a clear-cut idea on which food contains gluten. Part of this book is a list of ingredients you need to eliminate and another list for ingredients you can use to make the recipes. Label reading is also very essential in adopting this diet. Remember to check if the food is not manufactured or processed in the same plant that processed wheat products. Arm yourself with more knowledge about gluten and their sources so that you'd be able to identify their presence anytime, anywhere, easily. Be familiar with the funny names used by food manufacturers to conceal the gluten content in their food products. Strive to be a complete label reader.

When you're not sure, skip it. This should be your guiding principle always. It is always better to skip food; you are not sure contains gluten. Also, Be wary and vigilant of possible cross-contamination. Make sure the cooking vessels used to cook gluten loaded foodstuff were not used to prepare gluten-free meals.

Having a gluten-free diet is not all about restrictions and loss. This is also about abundance and variety and seeking ways to enjoying life. It doesn't mean that having no gluten will lead to no flavor, variety, or excitement. With some planning and creativity, you can still have the ability to indulge and enjoy your favorite comfort foods, even when having parties or going on a travel.

This book helped you embrace and live your gluten-free life to the fullest and help you reap the reward of long-term health through living gluten-free.

To end this book, I would like to take this opportunity once again to thank you for purchasing this book, and I hope that you found the content helpful! Here is wishing you a happy and healthy life!

Printed in Great Britain
by Amazon